The Implications of COVID-19 for Children and Youth

This book captures a unique moment in time, relatively early into the COVID-19 pandemic, when the implications and consequences of the pandemic remained unclear and largely unpredictable. The contributors to this volume contemplate the impact of the pandemic on our relationships with children and youth, child and youth serving systems, and broader issues in society that directly relate to childhood and youth. The essays collected in this volume cover a variety of perspectives that range from systemic racism in child-serving institutions to the politics of childhood during a pandemic, and the psychological and even neurological impacts of lockdowns, public restrictions, and social isolation. Beyond capturing the moment in time, the contributors also focused on the long term; they contemplated how the evolving situation might affect the way we think about child and youth services and our relationships to children, their families and their communities. From the very theoretical to the concrete and the practical, this volume provides current thinking and practice in relation to pandemic-impacted residential care settings, education and schools, hospital settings, communities, practitioners, and more.

This book was originally published as a special issue of the journal *Child & Youth Services.*

Grant Charles is a social work professor at the University of British Columbia, Vancouver, Canada, and the managing editor of *Child & Youth Services.*

Kiaras Gharabaghi is the dean of the Faculty of Community Services at Ryerson University, Toronto, Canada, and specializes in child and youth care practices locally and globally.

Shadan Hyder is a community activist and child and youth care practitioner in Toronto, Canada with a diploma, Bachelor and Masters degrees in Child and Youth Care.

Ashley Quinn is an Indigenous social work professor at the University of Toronto, Canada.

The Implications of COVID-19 for Children and Youth

Global Perspectives

Edited by

Grant Charles, Kiaras Gharabaghi, Shadan Hyder and Ashley Quinn

Routledge
Taylor & Francis Group
LONDON AND NEW YORK

First published 2023
by Routledge
4 Park Square, Milton Park, Abingdon, Oxon, OX14 4RN

and by Routledge
605 Third Avenue, New York, NY 10158

Routledge is an imprint of the Taylor & Francis Group, an informa business

British Library Cataloguing-in-Publication Data
A catalogue record for this book is available from the British Library

ISBN13: 978-1-032-22749-8 (hbk)
ISBN13: 978-1-032-22750-4 (pbk)
ISBN13: 978-1-003-27398-1 (ebk)

DOI: 10.4324/9781003273981

Typeset in Minion Pro
by codeMantra

Publisher's Note
The publisher accepts responsibility for any inconsistencies that may have arisen during the conversion of this book from journal articles to book chapters, namely the inclusion of journal terminology.

Contents

Citation Information

The chapters in this book were originally published in the journal *Child & Youth Services*, volume 41, issue 3 (2020). When citing this material, please use the original page numbering for each article, as follows:

Chapter 1
Editorial
Kiaras Gharabaghi, Shadan Hyder, Ashley Quinn, and Grant Charles
Child & Youth Services, volume 41, issue 3 (2020) pp. 205–207

Chapter 2
Disparities in Education: E-Learning and COVID-19, Who Matters?
Julet Allen, Fowzia Mahamed, and Ken Williams
Child & Youth Services, volume 41, issue 3 (2020) pp. 208–210

Chapter 3
CO-Vigilance: Radical Posturing for Uncertain Times
Peter Amponsah
Child & Youth Services, volume 41, issue 3 (2020) pp. 211–213

Chapter 4
Prop It up or Let It Fall? K-12 Schooling in and after COVID-19
Ben Anderson-Nathe
Child & Youth Services, volume 41, issue 3 (2020) pp. 214–218

Chapter 5
The Effects of COVID-19 Prevention Measures on Families
Jonathan Bailey and Johanne Jean-Pierre
Child & Youth Services, volume 41, issue 3 (2020) pp. 219–221

Chapter 6
Relationships between Human and Nonhuman Animals
Ranjana Basu
Child & Youth Services, volume 41, issue 3 (2020) pp. 222–224

Chapter 7
Leaving the Virus behind: Seeing the Glass Half Full Amidst COVID-19
Jeelu Susan Behanan
Child & Youth Services, volume 41, issue 3 (2020) pp. 225–227

Chapter 8
From Crisis to Opportunity: Rethinking Education in the Wake of COVID-19
Connie Bird and Hidesh Bhardwaj
Child & Youth Services, volume 41, issue 3 (2020) pp. 228–230

Chapter 9
The Distressing Levels of the Covid-19 Crisis
Jess Boon
Child & Youth Services, volume 41, issue 3 (2020) pp. 231–234

Chapter 10
Building Resilience in Covid-19
Andrea V. Breen and Heather Chalmers
Child & Youth Services, volume 41, issue 3 (2020) pp. 235–236

Chapter 11
Coronavirus Challenges for Family Social Workers in Hong Kong
Simon Chan
Child & Youth Services, volume 41, issue 3 (2020) pp. 237–239

Chapter 12
Reflections on Being Oppression-Adjacent in the Time of COVID
David Collins and Jeremy Christopher Kohomban
Child & Youth Services, volume 41, issue 3 (2020) pp. 240–245

Chapter 13
Social Protection: An Essential and Effective Social Policy Response During and After COVID-19
Julie L. Drolet
Child & Youth Services, volume 41, issue 3 (2020) pp. 246–249

Chapter 14
The Immanence of Change: Who Will Write the History of COVID-19?
Kiaras Gharabaghi
Child & Youth Services, volume 41, issue 3 (2020) pp. 250–252

Chapter 15
During a Pandemic, the Digital Divide, Racism and Social Class Collide: The Implications of COVID-19 for Black Students in High Schools
Sabrin Hassan and Beverly-Jean Daniel
Child & Youth Services, volume 41, issue 3 (2020) pp. 253–255

Chapter 16
Hiding and Being Found: How Inequity Found Its Spotlight during COVID-19 and What It Means for the Future
Joy Henderson
Child & Youth Services, volume 41, issue 3 (2020) pp. 256–258

Chapter 17
COVID-19 Pandemic and Public Private Partnerships: Supporting Children and Young People
Sydney Henry
Child & Youth Services, volume 41, issue 3 (2020) pp. 259–260

Chapter 18
Covid-19 and Vulnerable Families Living in Rural Locations: Building a System for Recovery
Rochelle Hine, Andrea Reupert, Phillip Tchernegovski, Jade Sheen, and Darryl Maybery
Child & Youth Services, volume 41, issue 3 (2020) pp. 261–265

Chapter 19
COVID 19: The Precarity of Families and Disability
Rachelle Hole and Tim Stainton
Child & Youth Services, volume 41, issue 3 (2020) pp. 266–268

Chapter 20
COVID-19 and Collective Grief
Shadan Hyder
Child & Youth Services, volume 41, issue 3 (2020) pp. 269–270

Chapter 21
COVID-19 in the Era of Opioid Overdose: A Glimmer of Hope in the Midst of Double Whammy Tragedy
Mohamed Ibrahim
Child & Youth Services, volume 41, issue 3 (2020) pp. 271–273

Chapter 22
Finding Our Power Together: Working with Indigenous Youth and Children during COVID-19
Nicole Ineese-Nash
Child & Youth Services, volume 41, issue 3 (2020) pp. 274–276

Chapter 23
Advocating for Health and Well-Being
Sara Jassemi
Child & Youth Services, volume 41, issue 3 (2020) pp. 277–279

Chapter 24
Covid-19 and Intergenerational Anxiety and Trauma
Cecilia M. Jevitt
Child & Youth Services, volume 41, issue 3 (2020) pp. 280–282

Chapter 25
The Longer-Term Ramifications of the Covid-19 Pandemic for Children, Families, and Their Communities
Daniel Ji and Grant Charles
Child & Youth Services, volume 41, issue 3 (2020) pp. 283–285

Chapter 26
The Crisis of Loss and Moral Injury – Lasting Effects of COVID-19 on Teenagers and Healthcare Workers
Richard La Fleur
Child & Youth Services, volume 41, issue 3 (2020) pp. 286–289

Chapter 27
COVID-19: Effects of the Shutdown on Children and Families in Child and Youth Care Services in Germany
Maya Lorch and Dunja Fuchs
Child & Youth Services, volume 41, issue 3 (2020) pp. 290–292

Chapter 28
Engagement Redefined: Children and Youth without parental Care during and post Covid-19, India
Kiran Modi and Leena Prasad
Child & Youth Services, volume 41, issue 3 (2020) pp. 293–295

Chapter 29
Covid: What's Next for Indigenous People?
Marie Nightbird
Child & Youth Services, volume 41, issue 3 (2020) pp. 296–298

Chapter 30
Challenges for Indigenous Children and Youth
Ashley Quinn
Child & Youth Services, volume 41, issue 3 (2020) pp. 299–300

Chapter 31
Covid-19 Fares Gently with Children and Youngsters, but They Bear a Large Burden Due to the Lock down of the Society
Charlotte Reedtz
Child & Youth Services, volume 41, issue 3 (2020) pp. 301–303

Chapter 32
COVID-19, the Opioid Epidemic and the Housing Crisis
Lydia Rezene
Child & Youth Services, volume 41, issue 3 (2020) pp. 304–306

Chapter 33
A Unique Experience
Jordan Risidore
Child & Youth Services, volume 41, issue 3 (2020) pp. 307–309

Chapter 34
COVID-19 and Youth in Detention
William Rowe
Child & Youth Services, volume 41, issue 3 (2020) pp. 310–312

Chapter 35
Renewed Grammars of Care: A(n Abbreviated) Case for the End of "the Service Provider"
Juanita Stephen and Nataleah Hunter-Young
Child & Youth Services, volume 41, issue 3 (2020) pp. 313–315

Chapter 36
Coronavirus and Youth
Curren Warf
Child & Youth Services, volume 41, issue 3 (2020) pp. 316–319

Chapter 37
Navigating the COVID-19 Pandemic: The Future of Children and Young People
Khadijah Williams
Child & Youth Services, volume 41, issue 3 (2020) pp. 320–322

Chapter 38
Galvanizing Solidarity Through Chaos: Policing, Surveillance and the Impact of COVID-19 on Black Canadian Youth
Keisha Evans and Lesa Francis
Child & Youth Services, volume 41, issue 3 (2020) pp. 323–326

Notes on Contributors

Julet Allen, Humber College and York University, Toronto, Canada.

Peter Amponsah, School of Social Work, York University, Toronto, Canada.

Ben Anderson-Nathe, Child and Family Studies, Portland State University, USA.

Jonathan Bailey, Faculty of Behavioural Sciences, Yorkville University, Fredericton, Canada.

Ranjana Basu, College of Interdisciplinary Studies, Royal Roads University, Victoria, Canada.

Jeelu Susan Behanan, Department of Social Work, Amrita Vishwa Vidyapeetham, Kollam, India.

Hidesh Bhardwaj, Werklund School of Education, University of Calgary, Canada.

Connie Bird, School of Social Work, University of British Columbia, Vancouver, Canada.

Jess Boon, Residential School History and Dialogue Centre, University of British Columbia Youth, Vancouver, Canada.

Andrea V. Breen, Department of Family Relations and Applied Nutrition, University of Guelph, Canada.

Heather Chalmers, Department of Child and Youth Studies, Brock University, St. Catharine's, Canada.

Simon Chan, Department of Social Work, Hong Kong Baptist University, Hong Kong, China.

Grant Charles, School of Social Work, University of British Columbia, Vancouver, Canada.

David Collins, The Children's Village, USA.

Julie L. Drolet, Faculty of Social Work (Central and Northern Alberta Region), University of Calgary, Edmonton, Canada.

Keisha Evans, University of Windsor, Ontario, Canada.

Lesa Francis, Black Legal Action Centre, Toronto, Canada.

Dunja Fuchs, Teacher of English, Geography, Religious, and Social Education, Berlin Spandau, Germany.

Kiaras Gharabaghi, Faculty of Community Services, Ryerson University, Toronto, Canada.

Sabrin Hassan, Factor-Inwentash Faculty of Social Work, University of Toronto, Canada.

Joy Henderson, Afro-Indigenous CYC working on CYC advocacy, Dip Assaulted Women and Children's Counsellor Advocate (AWCCA), Canada.

Sydney Henry, Village Academy (School of Agriculture), Watsonville, Jamaica.

Rochelle Hine, School of Rural Health, Monash University, Australia.

Rachelle Hole, Canadian Institute for Inclusion and Citizenship, University of British Columbia, Kelowna, Canada.

Nataleah Hunter-Young, York University, Toronto, Canada; Ryerson University, Toronto, Canada.

Shadan Hyder, Community Activist and Child and Youth Care Practitioner, Toronto, Canada.

Mohamed Ibrahim, School of Social Work, University of British Columbia, Vancouver, Canada.

Nicole Ineese-Nash, School of Child and Youth Care, Ryerson University, Toronto, Canada

Sara Jassemi, Division of Adolescent Health and Medicine, Department of Pediatrics, BC Children's Hospital and University of British Columbia, Vancouver, Canada.

Beverly-Jean Daniel, School of Child and Youth Care, Ryerson University, Toronto, Canada.

Johanne Jean-Pierre, School of Child and Youth Care, Ryerson University, Toronto, Canada.

Cecilia M. Jevitt, Department of Family Practice, Faculty of Medicine, University of British Columbia, Vancouver, Canada.

Daniel Ji, School of Social Work, University of British Columbia, Vancouver, Canada.

Jeremy Christopher Kohomban, The Children's Village, USA.

Richard La Fleur, Department of Psychology, University of West Georgia, Carrollton, USA.

Maya Lorch, Johannesstift Diakonie Youth Welfare Department, Educator in Residential Group for Children/Teenagers, Berlin, Germany.

Fowzia Mahamed, Toronto District School Board, Toronto, Canada.

Darryl Maybery, School of Rural Health, Monash University, Australia.

Kiran Modi, Udayan Care, Delhi, India.

Marie Nightbird, School of Social Work, University of British Columbia, Vancouver, Canada.

Leena Prasad, Udayan Care, Delhi, India.

Dr. William Rowe DSW, Professor Southern Connecticut State University, New Haven Connecticut.

Ashley Quinn, Indigenous Social Work, University of Toronto, Canada.

Charlotte Reedtz, Regional Centre for Child and Adolescent Mental Health and Child Welfare, The Arctic University of Norway-UiT, Tromsø, Norway.

Andrea Reupert, Faculty of Education, Monash University, Australia.

Lydia Rezene, Community Health Specialist, Toronto, Canada.

Jordan Risidore, Factor-Inwentash Faculty of Social Work, University of Toronto, Canada.

Jade Sheen, School of Psychology, Deakin University, Melbourne, Australia.

Tim Stainton, Canadian Institute for Inclusion and Citizenship, University of British Columbia, Kelowna, Canada.

Juanita Stephen, York University, Toronto, Canada.

Phillip Tchernegovski, Faculty of Education, Monash University, Australia.

Curren Warf, Department of Pediatrics, Division of Adolescent Health and Medicine, Faculty of Medicine, University of British Columbia, Vancouver, Canada.

Ken Williams, Youth and Family Supports, Toronto, Canada.

Khadijah Williams, Village Academy (School of Agriculture), Saint Ann, Jamaica.

Introduction

Our world changed dramatically in 2020. The spread of COVID-19 across all continents, in over 200 countries, in both urban and rural regions, has impacted virtually everyone and every aspect of social, cultural and economic activity. It has, of course, also impacted politically, potentially altering the course of incumbent governments' legitimacy crises on one end of the spectrum, or reelection prospects on the other end of the spectrum. Whether or not these impacts of the pandemic are permanent remains to be seen. Economies will likely recover eventually, people will go back to work, and the fundamental structures of societies will probably bounce back. But some things may well have changed permanently; first and foremost, this pandemic may indeed have changed the way we are together on this planet. From the seemingly mundane changes to how we greet each other – avoiding handshakes and kisses on the cheeks – to the obviously more substantive issues of how we trust each other, subtle movement toward new ways of being together is already becoming apparent. Perhaps just as importantly, 2020 will leave us with a new chapter in history; a chapter during which some rose to the challenge of the collective good, while others retreated to the protection of individual well-being and survival. We will remember each other's actions, non-actions, statements and positions. And, we will either choose to remember or choose to forget the sacrifices and important deeds of those who have kept many of us alive through their work – the health care workers, the grocery store clerks, the community workers. We designated them as heroes at the start of this crisis; notably, this language is quietly retreating, special wage increases of chronically underpaid workers are being rolled back, and state support programs for those most impacted by the crisis are nearing their end.

One of the more peculiar aspects of this crisis has been the impact on and the narrative about children and youth. Most crises, such as war, ecological disaster, and famine focus significantly on the impact on children and youth. This crisis, quite uniquely, really struggled with centering our usual victims. It turns out that just this once, children and youth appeared physically better equipped to fight the virus that has been killing especially the elderly by the hundreds of thousands. In many narratives about this crisis, children and youth have become weaponized – the virus infects them to no effect but they transfer it to the adults in their lives. Children and youth suddenly are dangerous, a threat to those in our societies accustomed to being in control.

We are putting together this Special Issue of Child & Youth Services because we wondered about how all of these shifts, movements and changes will impact the ways we are with children, youth, their families and their communities and the ways in which we will be with them post-pandemic. Many of those with a stake in this journal are professionals and academics who spend every day thinking about some aspect of being with children, youth, their families and their communities. And so we wonder: will anything have changed once this pandemic subsides? Will the wounds of contemporary society, exposed through the course of this pandemic, impact our relationships?

The wounds exposed are plentiful. In North America in particular, the pandemic has been accompanied by a renewed agitation related to police violence, anti-Black racism, and neo-colonial practices impacting disproportionately on equity-seeking communities. Fueled by the empirical data about racialized injustice in social sectors, in health care and in education laid bare through the pandemic, will there ever be trust in the relationships between white and racialized communities? Will young people recover from the potentially traumatic loss of grandparents and parents to the virus? Will adults recover from the pain of watching their parents die in old age homes, which, it turns out, are in many cases reflective of the worst of human indignity? Will professional social service workers reengage with communities that live in precarious, high-risk circumstance where the reemergence of infectious disease seems likely? Will we collectively be able to heal?

All of these are big questions with no certain answers. We will all have to wait and see. But in the meantime, we wanted to pose these kinds of questions to people with a stake in the future of our relationships with children, youth, their families and their communities. And so we did. Our editorial team of four includes: Dr. Grant Charles, a Social Work professor at the University of British Columbia and one of the managing Editors of this journal; Dr. Ashley Quinn, an Indigenous Social Work professor at the University of Toronto, Shadan Hyder, a community activist and child and youth care practitioner based in Toronto, and Dr. Kiaras Gharabaghi, a Professor of Child & Youth Care at Ryerson University in Toronto and formerly a Managing Editor of this journal. We asked the authors to provide their perspective on how we will be with children and youth, their families and communities, post-pandemic. We were determined to seek out people who can bring different wisdom, different experiences, different geographies to the table. Assembled in this Special Issue are the voices of very established academics and high-status professionals as well as the voices of students, of frontline community workers and those themselves deeply impacted by this pandemic. Our contributors identify with many communities, including Indigenous communities, Black communities, Muslim communities, LGBTQ2s + communities, disability communities and others. They have experience in health care sectors, community service sectors, education, universities, policy sectors and elsewhere. And they geographically represent urban centers and small towns in Canada, the United States, Germany, Hong Kong, Ghana, India, Jamaica, Australia and Norway.

We asked for short, reflective pieces of writing informed by both personal experience and professional or scholarly engagement. While we hoped for a direct engagement with the core question about future relations with children, youth, their families and communities, what we received in response varied. For many of our contributors, it is the here and now that needed to be addressed – both in positive ways that celebrate the creativity and the hard work of organizations and individuals to respond to this crisis, and in more critical ways that ask hard questions of longstanding and emerging social injustices, racisms, exclusions and marginalization. Other contributors were quick to move toward the future; they provide possibilities for what we might expect years down the road that are informed by a wide range of worldviews and perspectives. From the psychiatric lens to the on-going battle against racism, and from the challenges for traditional institutions such as schools to the opportunities for social innovators, our contributors have something to say about many possible scenarios. Their writing was subject to editorial review processes to ensure a quality of narrative commensurate with the journal's expectations, especially where English may not have been the first language of the author(s); and we also provided for a modified, external and blind peer review process, focused primarily on the internal consistency of arguments and the avoidance of empirical inaccuracies.

We present this Special Issue with considerable pride; these are difficult times for many people around the world, but there is comfort in knowing that many people are also thinking deeply about what we are facing now and where we might find opportunities to make positive and meaningful change. Some contributions end on hopeful notes; others provide for clear and unequivocal warnings that we are in deep trouble as a human collective. Regardless, collectively these contributions give us a sense of possibilities, and that is in and of itself invaluable at a time of great uncertainty.

Kiaras Gharabaghi

Shadan Hyder

Ashley Quinn

Grant Charles

Disparities in Education: E-Learning and COVID-19, Who Matters?

Julet Allen, Fowzia Mahamed, and Ken Williams

A great deal of attention during this pandemic has been placed on health disparities; however, the educational inequities become apparent in how emergency remote learning reinforces educational inequities for Black students. This crisis has highlighted cracks in the education system that have always existed, including inequitable access with respect to e-learning as a mode of instruction.

Between 1995 and 2003, the Ontario education policy underwent significant reforms during the “Common Sense Revolution” (CSR) years of Mike Harris’s Conservative government. The rationalization for restructuring was to improve outcomes and ensure accountability to remain globally competitive in a market-driven economy (Basu, 2004). Prior to these changes in 1993, Ontario’s first social-democratic government led by Bob Rae developed and started to implemented anti-racism and ethnocultural equity policies structured as a systemic policy approach to educational equity; however, these approaches were abandoned when the Conservatives came to power.

Before COVID-19, there had been a steady push by Black researchers and the community for the collection of race base data in education. Failure by governments to collect data based on race limits how educational outcomes are examined for Black students (Robson, 2018). Race-based data collection on e-learning is needed to examine how Black students will fare, especially in this time of the pandemic, when they continue to face multiple barriers. The students who thrive at e-learning are those who are concentrated in the most privileged schools in the city and are identified by the Toronto District School Board (TDSB) as having higher learning opportunities (Farhadi, 2019). Black learners often reside in communities fraught with socioeconomic, social, political and educational disparities and they do not always have access to multiple devices, broadband internet and parents who can work from home. Instead, they face higher rates of poverty, overcrowded households and parents with the inability to work from home as Black peoples are over-represented in front-line positions.

E-learning, when happening outside of a pandemic, takes away 440 h of face-to-face-class time, which can intensify disparities in access in an education system already fraught with systemic anti-Black racism (Farhadi, 2019). The adoption of e-learning is not recommended because it risks contributing to and reinforcing inequitable education policies as it fails to acknowledge race and discrimination which are factors seldom measured and addressed. When she was the Minister of Education in Ontario, Lisa Thompson, queried the question of "What's wrong with our student's embracing technology?" As great as she imagined this progress in education, she simply overlooked the complex issues the education system poses for many students, especially those living on the margins. With an education system steeped in anti-Black racism, the collection of race-based data would capture how many Black students have inadequate resources to be successful with e-learning platforms and what percentage of Black students will attain the educational outcomes for 2020.

The lack of race-base data collection stems from the notion that Canada is a "colour-blind" society, therefore, there is no racism and that racism is something that occurs south of the border (Robson, 2018). The systems under which we operate are not "colour-blind," and doing nothing will leave inequities unaddressed (Gawley, 2020). Research coming from the United States and the United Kingdom identifies that Black peoples and communities have been affected by the virus at an alarming rate. If Canada continues to proceed and not consider the collection of educational race-based data during the pandemic, it leaves us with the inability to develop public policies to respond to the needs of those most vulnerable and marginalized. The failure of the government to collect this data will reinforce the historic and current impacts of colonial violence and continued systemic inequities (Timothy, 2020).

Njoki Wane (2020) suggests that Canadians have a deep attachment to principles of equity that is associated with the belief that all individuals, regardless of ethnicity, race, and religion are rewarded solely based on merit. However, meritocracy is a myth and a dangerous ally to neoliberal ideology that disavows systemic structures of oppression that are built within institutions such as the education system. Neoliberalism has re-articulated the meaning of equity and justice in education and created a system of winners and losers, and these policies legitimize losing as solely an individual failing (Rezai-Rashti et al., 2017).

Black and racialized students are replaced with "at-risk" labels or "recent immigrant" status; this further reduces their visibility and highlights the underachievement gaps these policies are trying to address. Black lives continue not to matter. E-learning amplifies these inequities among Black students who face a plethora of challenges, such as low academic achievements and a sense of unworthiness within Canadian society as a whole.

References

Basu, R. (2004). The rationalization of neoliberalism in Ontario's public education system, 1995-2000. *Geoforum*, *35*(5), 621–634. https://doi.org/10.1016/j.geoforum.2004.03.003

Farhadi, B. (2019, October 17). In Doug Ford's e-learning gamble, high school students will lose. *The Conversation*. https://theconversation.com/in-doug-fords-e-learning-gamble-high-school-students-will-lose-122826

Gawley, K. (2020, April 7). Canada's 'colourblind' coronavirus data could leave officials blind to racial inequities. *City News*. https://www.citynews1130.com/2020/04/07/canadas-colourblind-coronavirus-data-could-leave-officials-blind-to-racial-inequities/

Rezai-Rashti, G., Segeren, A., & Martino, W. (2017). The new articulation of equity education in neoliberal times: The changing conception of social justice in Ontario. *Globalisation, Societies and Education*, *15*(2), 160–174. https://doi.org/10.1080/14767724.2016.1169514

Robson, K. (2018, December 12). Why won't Canada collect data on race and student success? *Brighter World, McMaster University*. https://brighterworld.mcmaster.ca/articles/why-wont-canada-collect-data-on-race-and-student-success/

Timothy, R. K. (2020, April 6). Coronavirus is not the great equalizer-race matters. *The Conversation*. https://theconversation.com/coronavirus-is-not-the-great-equalizer-race-matters-133867

Wane, N. (2020). Experiences of visible minority students and anti-racist education within the Canadian education system. *Journal of Thought*, *39*(1), 25–44.

CO-Vigilance: Radical Posturing for Uncertain Times

Peter Amponsah

What a time to be alive. We have entered the 21st year of the 21st century. Scientists have declared these times the Anthropocene (Steffen et al., 2018); a new geological epoch that marks humanity's impact on the Earth. We now have the language to help us understand the rise in sea levels and CO_2 emissions, fluctuating weather conditions and the mass extinction of plant life and species. Our social infrastructure is weak; from social security, to healthcare, to systems of care for the young and old, the weight of human need seems to have surpassed human ingenuity. According to the World Health Organization (2020), this never seen before coronavirus has killed hundreds of thousands of people and crippled global economies and necessarily shrunk our personal, collective, and regional boundaries. Distance learning and work from home have crossed boundaries, becoming the new normal, morphing our days and nights into a single block of time. Self-reflection and self-discovery have become their own brands, while inaction and apathy lurks silently in our sleepless nights. All the while, young lives… young Black bodies, their hopes and dreams, continue to be jeopardized at the hands of hate-fuelled racism.

Vigilance is an act or state of keeping careful watch for possible danger, threats, or difficulties. For those of us who live, play, work with and/or care for children, youth and their families, and communities, the context that these times provide is an opportunity for observation and on-going opposition to those seeking to protect the status quo by defining and dictating our human response to our current crisis. Far from the status quo, what we really need is a CO-vigilant stance. A heightened sensitivity that would help to avoid being entrapped by the politic and emotions of the day. Such a stance grapples with the inescapable reality that Black and racialized communities are the most impacted in any crisis, COVID-19 further confirming this.

The greatest (and most destructive) impacts of COVID-19 are borne by Black bodies, but this remains largely invisible to the masses already fully engaged in the 'public health narrative' presenting this crisis as universal.

We have observed the re-deployment of the term essential worker, a designation that in its current use disguises the perfunctory nature of anti-Black racism by shifting value and recognition between bodies and function. Rather, it is those whose essential work, a majority of them Black and racialized bodies, who have had to tend to the care of the most vulnerable populations throughout this time. This is significant, because in the face of danger and fear, these individuals have shown that the role of caregiver and the responsibility and resolve to care, has the potential to not only neutralize uncertainty, but also to uphold, strengthen and protect humanity and human dignity. This is also significant because care and caregiving are not individualistic concepts, notwithstanding the desire of our hero-culture to render them as such. In fact, care and caregiving transcends the individual's activity and involves additionally a transference in Black and racialized families and communities when frontline workers bring their fear home. A contagion of despair, so insidious that without clear articulation goes dismissed.

Let's consider this, when young Black people bare witness to Black bodies being infected by COVID-19 in greater numbers, white privilege continues to exert itself through ease of access to medical, social, and economic protection. Why then is the mere suggestion to governments to move from the anecdotal to the factual in order to understand the place of race met with political agitation, tactical avoidance and rapid change of topic? It is in this context that we find ourselves battling a human crisis of epic proportion.

I have heard that out of despair springs hope, an interesting conceptualization when one considers the scale of global despair taking place. What might this mean for our work with young people going forward, particularly those whose faces reflect the caregivers, the sick, and the dead? For one, the metaphorical shedding of social debris through pause and reflection during this time has provided a tabula rasa of sorts for child and youth care work. Our next iterations of theory and practice must transcend our reliance on organizations, institutions and infrastructure in addressing the physical safety and wellbeing of children and youth. These entities, tied to the politics of privilege and whiteness, have context and time-limited presence in young people's lives and have proven themselves not reliable even in moments of stability; they certainly have failed miserably during the current moment of instability, and one can expect them to fail again the next time we face such a moment. We need to care for the minds of our young; the bombardment of risk discourses deployed in this current moment has the potential to re-edify the confining practices of our past; an anti-liberatory practice that would rather have us clinging onto oppressive traditions instead of innovation. We require a posturing that is not only concerned with the specific outcomes of inequity, but also the historical circumstances and ruling relations that provide the conditions in which Child and Youth Care unfolds now and has always existed.

The vigilance of this moment is likely to carry forward into post-COVID times. This is unfortunate, because this vigilance is based on fear, risk avoidance, and a reliance on distant expertise gained in the mysterious halls of science and exclusive institutions of higher (and privileged) knowledge. This is the vigilance of whiteness, seemingly appropriate in the response to a threatening virus, but quite comfortable in its acceptance of the collateral damage, which includes the disproportionate dying of Black and racialized peoples. We cannot afford vigilance; we must strive toward CO-vigilance, and begin to articulate fears and opportunities, care and protection, individual safety, and community well-being such that we explicitly and directly acknowledge and act upon the many ways that longstanding and chronically entrenched inequities and racisms render this moment not a public health crisis, but a well-deserved spiritual crisis for the privileged soul. As we look to what is next for Child and Youth Care, we should never forget that young people and their caregivers are the cornerstone of our future. For this future to be different, for it to be better, young people, including Black and racialized young people as well as their caregivers, must have experiences of mattering, of being valued as essential, now.

References

Steffen, W., Rockström, J., Richardson, K., Lenton, T. M., Folke, C., Liverman, D., Summerhayes, C. P., Barnosky, A. D., Cornell, S. E., Crucifix, M., Donges, J. F., Fetzer, I., Lade, S. J., Scheffer, M., Winkelmann, R., & Schellnhuber, H. J. (2018). Trajectories of the earth system in the anthropocene. *Proceedings of the National Academy of Sciences of the United States of America*, *115*(33), 8252–8259. https://doi.org/10.1073/pnas.1810141115

World Health Organization. (2020). *Coronavirus disease (COVID-19) outbreak situation*. https://www.who.int/emergencies/diseases/novel-coronavirus-2019.

Prop It up or Let It Fall? K-12 Schooling in and after COVID-19

Ben Anderson-Nathe

The COVID-19 moment is one of uncertainty and vulnerability, across all sectors and populations. Even as many countries are gradually re-opening, we see infection rates continuing to rise and anticipate second and third waves of infection in the coming months. Reactions to this moment vary widely, but as can be expected in times of such uncertainty, anxieties are high. Precarity is the name of the game, made worse by systemic inequities of racism, poverty, capitalism, xenophobia, and more. As many people look to familiar institutions for comfort and stability, the pandemic is exposing those institutions' fundamental fragility. Compulsory, benchmarked, age-segregated K-12 schooling is one such institution rocked by its own fragility.

In the United States, educational inequities have been amply documented. We have a public education system in which very few really thrive, many make do, and many experience school as primarily a site of exclusion, isolation, or failure. That these experiences are organized along clear dimensions of race, class, gender, and (dis)ability has been well documented. Even still, for many young people in the US–even those who may not experience schools as sites of learning or affirmation–the school remains a safe(r) place than their homes. US schools provide supervision, food, shelter during the school day, health care services, and more; for many, they are an essential feature of an already compromised social safety net. For children living in abusive contexts, schools and their staff are often first responders and young people's primary source of support. In recent weeks, child welfare reports have fallen far below average, which suggests not that children are no longer being abused, but that in many cases they have lost contact with supportive adults who may at other times have noticed and sought help.

As social distancing closed brick-and-mortar schools, (relatively) much was made in the public arena about the ways in which students who rely on schools for these services would suffer. Schools created mechanisms for families to access meals and other services. Equity advocates pointed out the obvious issues of access to technology and connectivity that would prevent some students (again, largely along raced and classed lines) from accessing schooling in its new 'home-based learning' format. So districts across the country mobilized, redirected funds, and sought to provide tablets to every family and even help offset the cost of internet service. And these strategies are good, as far as they go.

With the rhetoric in place that districts had provided access, March and April saw a full-steam-ahead approach to home based learning, which positioned parents as their children's teachers, and children as their parents' students. Social media was abuzz with home-learning schedules and innovative lesson plans provided by these parents who had now become teachers. Online education platforms and curriculum marketers have expanded access to their materials to help students stay 'on track'. A clear social expectation has emerged: it is now the responsibility of parents to see to it that their children would not 'fall behind'. Parents have been expected to preside over their children's Zoom sessions, to teach 'the new math' that they themselves were never taught. And children are expected to fall in line and perform at home as they had performed at school.

There are, of course, many problems with this orientation. First, it presumes that parents had the flexibility to take on this new role–again, an assumption that largely plays out in predictably classed and raced ways. Second, it presumes that parents had the skill to take on this new role, which many simply did not. Third, it presumes that all students could simply make this transition, that young people learn equally well in online settings, and that instruction for students with disabilities could be reasonably accommodated at home, with few supports, and no formal training for parents. Finally, and perhaps most significantly, it presumes that schooling is the most important feature of a young person's life. The role of 'student' in this COVID moment has become young people's central role, even to the extent that their parents' roles have shifted to accommodate it.

These observations raise at least two additional dilemmas that have received much less discussion in the public sphere. One concerns the disruptions to family roles and parent-child relationships as parents become their children's educators and children become their parents' pupils. For young people whose experiences of schooling have been largely affirmative, it might stand to reason that this role transition could roll out smoothly. If education is a context in which young people feel good about themselves, participating in lessons at home may produce few adverse effects beyond possibly boredom at the tasks. But for children whose school lives have sent a message of exclusion or failure–for those who have been consistently told by school that they are 'behind,' that they are problematic, that they simply can't learn–transferring the school environment to the home, and the relationship between student and teacher to child and parent, has more dire consequences.

In this case, parents' ability to buffer the strain of children's transition to this new COVID world is compromised by those same parents' newfound responsibility to deliver the educational experience. The parent becomes the teacher, and in taking on that role also takes on the child's response to that role. The result? Increased strain among families, role confusion at a time when the social order itself is inconsistent and unpredictable, and reinforcement of children's negative associations with the educational experience. If we have learned anything from family systems theory and theories of families, stress, and change, we know the strain such disequilibrium produces for systems as roles shift and family patterns are interrupted. And amid these strains, most families' access to the resources (emotional, material, financial) to respond to stress are at an all-time low. In such circumstances, it is difficult to conceive of much academic learning occurring.

The other dilemma speaks to the fragility of an education system rooted in age-graded and segregated schooling wedded to standardized benchmarking that renders some young people 'on track' while others are positioned either 'ahead' or 'behind.' The social expectation that formal schooling continue in the pandemic, and the shifted burden of that schooling to individual families, has forced parents to divert their attention from their children's (mental, emotional, and physical) responses to a generation-defining moment, to their performance against arbitrary academic expectations. Many parents have received messages, from schools and even more insidiously from one another, that to be 'good' parents in this moment means providing 'good' educational structures for children to learn from home. Their worries are echoed by their children's teachers: 'How will my child be ready for the next grade in the fall?' 'How far behind will my child be?' 'What do I need to do now so my child keeps up with their grade level?' These questions, while well intentioned, miss the point.

Grades and standards and benchmarks have no enduring meaning by themselves. They take significance only when we agree they are significant. What makes someone 'ready' for fourth grade? Only the predetermined agreement that they must have accomplished x, y, and z in third grade. There is no universal or *a priori* set of knowledge or skills that children must know at age nine in order to be prepared for age ten. This point is driven home when we realize that these standards shift every few years. In many states, Kindergarteners are now expected to read by the end of the year; in previous educational moments, this first year of schooling focused almost entirely on social and emotional learning. There is an opportunity in the COVID moment to recognize that grade-based benchmarks are, for the most part, arbitrary. Some children will meet them, and others will not.

This is likely to be as much due to children's history with schooling and the messages they've received about themselves as it does with actual learning. It is related as much to families' experiences living through or dying amid this pandemic as it is to mastery of, say, fifth grade content. To reinforce aspirations or expectations that parents act as proxies for teachers, that videoconferences stand in for classrooms, and that children perform to educational expectations as though everything else was normal is to underscore the educational inequities we know exist even in the best of times. Those children who are already doing just fine will likely continue to do fine. And those who are not? They will suffer even more.

So, to the central question of this Special Issue: What are the ramifications of this moment for children and families? First, we must recognize that this moment is without precedent. None of our previous ways of relating work the way they used to, and they're not likely to return to normal even once a vaccine is available and social distancing guidelines relax. And we should be wary of the nostalgia trap, falling into a misperception that 'normal' was working in the first place. Second, we need to affirm that this moment will in fact define generations. Just as children of the Great Depression carried fears of scarcity with them into adulthood, children and youth today will carry lessons we have not yet conceptualized into their tomorrows as well. And finally, we can hear the call to attend to these realities with and for children, observing how they process this moment, what questions arise for them, what nameless fears send them crying into their bedrooms. We can recognize that in a moment of heightened anxiety, those children whose relationships to school are already precarious will experience even more vulnerability.

This leads me to believe we have two options as we end the 2019–20 school year. One option is to proceed as though schooling in the fall will go back to normal. Children will advance a grade and will be benchmarked again in September against standardized assessments, and they will be sorted into advanced, at grade level, or remedial learners. And we can predict with great clarity, I'm sure, which children will be sorted where. This option is easy, in some ways, because it requires little disruption in a status quo. But it belies our stated rhetoric that education is a right and our school systems are committed to equity in that education. To choose this option demands a reckoning with hypocrisy of that rhetoric.

A second option is more radical, but also in my view more humane, more equitable, and more ethical. We can stop propping up an educational structure that sorts children based on arbitrary age-graded markers of achievement. We can recognize that the COVID moment means nothing will be like it was before, and in that recognition, we can seize the opportunity to remake education. We can take a note from special education's cardinal principal of differentiated instruction. We can say to children, and to families, that it is more important in the moment to process and make sense of this pandemic–its grief and loss, its uncertainty, its profound and prolonged disequilibrium–than it is to perform 'good studenthood' or 'good parent-teacherhood.' And to be fair, some schools–such as my own child's–have approached the COVID moment in this spirit. I have no clear vision of just what this transformed educational system may look like in the long run, being a product of it my whole life. But I believe it is possible that the pandemic may provide a window through which we can envision something different for our schools, that centers actual young people and holistic learning. To do anything else, while certainly easier, is to knowingly leave behind the most vulnerable children, youth, and families.

The Effects of COVID-19 Prevention Measures on Families

Jonathan Bailey and Johanne Jean-Pierre

The COVID-19 pandemic will have short- and long-term effects on families. We believe that the closure of schools puts parents in a precarious position to assume several additional roles and responsibilities. In addition, the loss of access to community services and cultural institutions has a disproportionate negative effect on marginalized families.

Prior to the Covid-19 pandemic, support systems for families spanned a wide range of institutions and community services. Families were able to determine their own level of participation in available supports to maintain or improve family functioning and child and youth success. However, the ongoing pandemic and the global response to curtailing its effects is proving to have significant consequences on children, youth, and families (Kury de Castillo, 2020). The necessity to self-isolate and engage in social distancing has resulted in the loss of social interactions and child development opportunities outside of the family home.

Because it is a place where resources and learning opportunities can be shared with all students, several authors have suggested that the contemporary school may in fact contribute to reduce inequalities and, in many ways, equalize access to key developmental and educational resources for students from disadvantaged backgrounds (Cebolla-Boado et al., 2017; von Hippel et al., 2018). In the short-term, due to the closure of schools to prevent the spread of COVID-19, nearly all families have lost access to the primary resource for their children to receive formal learning, socialization, and various forms of developmental, social and cultural stimulation. This translates into a loss of key social ties in the form of teachers, educational assistants, peers, and other professionals such as counselors, social workers, and psychologists. It is understandably overwhelming for parents, on such short notice and with little time to prepare, to adopt the role of an all-encompassing support for their children while they attempt to engage in home-schooling combined with tele-work or employment insecurity.

In addition to the closure of schools, families are also unable to access critical community services and cultural institutions that usually serve as additional or complementary individual and collective forms of support. Families are unable to attend cultural, linguistic, religious, or spiritual-specific activities that may have great significance for identity formation and the sense of belonging of children, youth and families (Etter et al., 2019; King et al., 2011; Nortier, 2018). In addition, recreational, athletic, and artistic activities are out of reach but are known to have a positive impact on child and youth development (Oftedal & Schneider, 2013). Members of marginalized communities tend to rely more strongly on community resources, as they can contribute to mental health and wellbeing, can be culturally relevant, and can enable civic engagement within their own communities. Many households depend on external educational, social, and cultural community resources to achieve their family aspirations and improve their overall wellbeing. With these sources unavailable to them, marginalized families and children are likely experiencing high levels of stress in addition to what the general population is exposed to.

While the long-term consequences of COVID-19 prevention measures are uncertain, gradual deconfinement measures will result in a return to school, work, community gatherings, and public events. Families and communities are resilient and are only required to wait until this pandemic passes to reconnect with community members and peers. The ability of families to recover from the long-term consequences of the pandemic, however, will largely depend on access to key resources. These resources include access to employment to increase financial security and schools to provide formal learning. In addition, community members, professionals, and not-for-profit organization staff will work with parents to bridge important gaps and provide tailored interventions.

An important caveat to these assumptions of the short- and long-term recovery from the pandemic for families is the ability of governments to support community services. Marginalized families disproportionately use community services (Kidd & McKenzie, 2014) as supports and will require access that corresponds to their needs to achieve a semblance of return to a normal life. We can only hope that adequate funding will be directed to various educational, community, and cultural institutions in order to maintain an optimal level of resources for all the families that can benefit from supports.

The reintroduction of these resources after the lockdowns will need to be paired with tremendous efforts by professionals to work closely with the children, youth, and families who once relied on them. Workers must establish and adopt new safety protocols in order to best serve their communities and to present a welcoming environment for the community's return. Time and an acknowledgement of community concerns will allow past relationships to reconnect and build toward a new future.

ORCID

Jonathan Bailey http://orcid.org/0000-0002-6676-5001
Johanne Jean-Pierre http://orcid.org/0000-0003-4451-7098

References

Cebolla-Boado, H., Radl, J., & Salazar, L. (2017). Preschool education as the great equalizer? A cross-country study into the sources of inequality in reading competence. *Acta Sociologica*, *60*(1), 41–60. https://doi.org/10.1177/0001699316654529

Etter, M., Goose, A., Nossa, M., Chishom-Nelson, J., Heck, C., Joober, R., Boksa, P., Lal, S., Shah, J. L., Andersson, N., Iyer, S. N., & Malla, A. (2019). Improving youth mental wellness services in an Indigenous context in Ulukhaktok, Northwest Territories: ACCESS Open Minds Project. *Early Intervention in Psychiatry*, *13*(S1), 35–41. https://doi.org/10.1111/eip.12816

Kidd, S., & McKenzie, K. (2014). Social entrepreneurship and services for marginalized groups. *Ethnicity and Inequalities in Health and Social Care*, *7*(1), 3–13. https://doi.org/10.1108/EIHSC-03-2013-0004

King, P. E., Carr, D., & Boitor, C. (2011). Religion, spirituality, positive youth development, and thriving. *Advances in Child Development and Behavior*, *41*, 161–195. https://doi.org/10.1016/B978-0-12-386492-5.00007-5

Kury de Castillo, C. (2020, April). *It's very stressful': Parents struggle with teaching children at home through COVID-19*. Global News.

Nortier, J. (2018). Language and identity practices among multilingual Western European youths. *Language and Linguistics Compass*, *12*(5), e12278. https://doi.org/10.1111/lnc3.12278

Oftedal, A., & Schneider, I. E. (2013). Outdoor recreation availability, physical activity, and health outcomes: County-level analysis in Minnesota. *Journal of Park and Recreation Administration*, *31*(1), 34–56.

von Hippel, P. T., Workman, J., & Downey, D. B. (2018). Inequality in reading and math skills forms mainly before kindergarten: A replication, and partial correction, of "Are schools the great equalizer?" *Sociology of Education*, *91*(4), 323–357. https://doi.org/10.1177/0038040718801760

Relationships between Human and Nonhuman Animals

Ranjana Basu

I am especially interested in our relationships with nonhuman animals. I use this term to highlight that humans are animals too. Now that I've done so, I'll refer to nonhuman animals as animals in this article. Many children, youth, and families have strong bonds with companion animals. Many other animals share space with us in our communities, and we encounter some daily and others only when we wander in the wilderness. What has this coronavirus pandemic meant for and about our relationship with all these beings and how has that affected us?

Families staying at home means spending more time together and more interaction between human and nonhuman family members. When we go for walks with our dog, my husband and I have noticed many more people walking with their dogs than before COVID-19. This seems to be good for both species because they are getting exercise, enjoying each other's company, and neighbors have an opportunity to speak briefly with each other from across the street. As we know, though, being at home is not a safe place for everyone. Companion animals are known to be a support to vulnerable members of a family, so I imagine this role is even more important now. For vulnerable companion animals, having additional nonabusive family members at home also provides some buffer. Animal abuse and family violence co-occur with a host of serious harms suffered by human (all ages) and animal family members, and these situations have been intensified with the relentless proximity to perpetrator(s) caused by the COVID-19 stay-at-home measures. I am concerned about the wellbeing of all vulnerable individuals — human and animal — at home. We need to help them stay safe, and I hope this pandemic is forcing us to think of new ways of doing so.

There have been reports in the news of wild animals that live in our communities coming out of hiding to walk the streets now that people are staying in. It's a reminder that these animals share our space. Yet we do not acknowledge them as community members and rarely contemplate how we may cohabitate. Rather, we recognize them mainly when we come into conflict and then our primary goal is to be rid of the nuisance. We are so focused on our desires that we generally do not consider their needs. Why should we since they are not like us? Does this kind of thinking sound familiar? Isn't this how a dominant group marginalizes minority groups who are different from them? Of course, there is one fundamental difference: They are animals and we are humans after all! But I started this opinion piece pointing out that humans are animals too. So what makes us so special? The standard that we require nonhuman animals to meet to be granted moral status keeps changing as we find out more and more about what different animals are capable of. The point here is that our exceptional status is a social construction. Yes, we are different, but this is not surprising. All species of animals are different from each other as are individuals within each species. There are also similarities. Being different, though, is not a reason to devalue another.

How we value and treat animals is related to how we value and treat each other in our families, communities, and beyond. This pandemic gives us good reason to scrutinize this. There have been reports that the COVID-19 spread originated in so-called "wet" markets. This is a euphemistic term for markets where live animals are killed, and their dead body parts sold directly to consumers for food. The jump of a pathogen from animal to human or vice versa can cause what is called a zoonotic disease, a term with which we are becoming increasingly familiar. The World Health Organization tells us that the SARS and Ebola viruses are thought to have originated in bats, and that evidence suggests the dromedary camel in the Middle East are reservoirs for the transmission of the Middle East Respiratory Syndrome-CoV. Dr. Jane Goodall recently explained that zoonotic diseases from wild animals are more prevalent now because the destruction of their habitats for land development and animal agriculture has resulted in animals having less space. This causes animals to live in closer proximity to each other as well as to humans. This proximity increases the chances of contact through which disease can spread. Furthermore, factory farms, in which *billions* of animals are grown and killed *annually* for food, are a recognized source of antibiotic-resistant bacteria that can infect humans. They are transmitted through the consumption of meat. The millions of tonnes of waste and methane gas produced from these sordid farms, where animals are forcefully crammed together in unhygienic conditions, pollute our soil and waterways and result in more greenhouse gas emissions than the world's entire automobile industry. How we treat animals, then, is related to our public health.

COVID-19 is yet another harsh reminder that we are connected to the other beings who live on this planet and to the land, water, and air we share. It is a reminder to think seriously about our relations with animals, each other, and our surroundings. Amidst the shutdown of almost all that we know about how our society functions, I've been thinking about creating a different future when *this* pandemic has passed, starting now. Our relationships with animals are a central part of this. I'm imagining we will pay more attention and treat all of *us* (not *us* and *them*) with respect. We will stop the tremendous "necessary" harms we inflict on other animals. We will see that the oppression of animals and humans is connected and therefore all are important, an understanding illuminated by feminist intersectional analysis. To change the present trajectory, we have to *think* and *do* differently at all levels of analysis. Otherwise we can expect more of the same.

Leaving the Virus Behind: Seeing the Glass Half Full Amidst COVID-19

Jeelu Susan Behanan

We are going through an unusual situation. During this pandemic, when India has been under lockdown for what seems like a very long time, the impact on children, families, and communities is interesting to think about. Though the pandemic has brought a lot of worries, deaths, loss, and uncertainties, let us still try to see the glass half full. With all our efforts to stop the transmission of the virus, we have to move forward and not be bound to this season of life.

Adapting to massive and far-reaching change is challenging and often takes time. The lockdown imposed in India is an unprecedented approach to deal with a crisis in this country and this extreme measure has not been easy for a population who thrives on social and cultural engagement. For some people, the loss of structure and routine in daily life has been experienced as extremely challenging; for others, the time at home and with immediate family allowed for more time for balancing all domains of life. People could not follow all the protocols initially and there were a lot of violations reported. Notably, however, people started to be more hygienic, especially performing hand hygiene and taking time for self-care. If people try to carry these positive aspects of this shift in lifestyle further, there will be a significant gain from the pandemic.

Gradually, people are adapting to the circumstances presenting themselves at the moment. They have found surprising ways of making use of the unexpected extra time spent at home. There are no more family get-togethers and ceremonial functions, but within families, there is more time for fun, creativity, care, and togetherness. What children did alone before, they now do with their parents, thereby cultivating a space for the growth and development of children with enough environmental stimulation, as well as the growth of relational connectedness within (often multi-generational) family units.

None of this has been easy for either the children or the parents. The temptation to put a mobile into the child's hands is great, as this would make it easier for parents to do their work. But, that's not always ideal because parent–child interactions and their attentiveness to the said and unsaid needs of children do play a vital role in the kind of attachment children develop. For children and youth, it is not easy to stay away from their playmates or social outings, but there is joy in rediscovering that the family is not as boring as anticipated when there is sufficient collective effort to generate friendship, joy, and attention. Beyond the parents, the newfound turn toward family also impacts the elder generations who often form part of the household. We know that the elderly are at higher risk, not only of infection but also of mental health concerns brought on by loneliness and isolation. As a result, many elderly people value the lockdown phase for giving their children and grandchildren some extra time at home. This pandemic has given more time to individuals of all ages to share all those triumphant stories, childhood memories, and hardships that are embedded in the lives of the different generations.

This pandemic provides us with an opportunity to think and act beyond our immediate premises, our households, and our families. In reality, our lives are interdependent, and what lies beyond our immediate physical context, the communities all around us, are our true neighborhood. The planet has witnessed a lot of ups and downs, fighting between races and religions, discrimination based on sexuality and gender and abuses of power. India is no stranger to these kinds of human failings, but neither are the countries of the Global North, where the virus and the consequences of responding to the virus as a public health threat disproportionately impact some population groups. We have learned through these experiences that these longstanding battles between privilege and marginality are not at all helpful in the global fight against this virus. The virus is entirely unmoved by the battles we fight against one another. We can see here in India and everywhere else in the world that the time to move beyond these battles is now. Discrimination, oppression, marginalization, and exclusion, on whatever basis, can now be readily labeled as globally counterproductive. One possible outcome of this crisis may be that we learn to act together, as a global village. Being with children, youth, families, and communities post-COVID means learning the hard lessons the pandemic is teaching. Collective spirit and action, inclusion and embrace, giving where possible rather than taking when available, are the new ways in which we must learn to be with others generally, but especially with those most vulnerable.

At times, all we can see is the glass half empty. There is a good reason for that. The experiences of people during this pandemic vary significantly. Again, this is true in India as much as it is true anywhere else. The experiences of service providers like health professionals, police officers, people working in media, and volunteers providing care to others surely are characterized by many more challenges. These people are involved in the provision of care at great risk to themselves. They might barely have time for family or even for themselves, and whatever time they do have to come together with loved ones is overshadowed by the knowledge of a heightened risk of infection. To live under the threat of being diagnosed is suffocating. The very idea of social isolation is devastating for people whose lives are dependent on social supports and contacts, such as the elderly, the poor, the marginalized, and the homeless. In contemplating the glass half full, we must be careful not to trivialize or minimize the sacrifices and sufferings of our fellow beings who are experiencing the worst of this pandemic now and who will likely continue to experience challenges long after this pandemic has passed.

At a time when people are getting sick and many are dying, it is difficult to contemplate a post-COVID world. There are no clear responses to our uncertainties as of yet. In seeing the glass half full, we cautiously but optimistically calculate the long-term impact of increased family engagement unfolding now. Interactions within a family, peer group, society or any context is an essential component that enhances the quality of culture, collective spirit, and togetherness. The way we will be with children, youth, and families moving forward will hopefully be based on the positive developmental and attachment effects of parents playfully touching their children more during their confinements at home; perhaps also by the therapeutic touch of nurses to the patient in care. Touch in this case is a metaphor for all that we give and for a newfound sense of connectedness. Notwithstanding the enormous challenges associated with COVID-19, we may come out of this pandemic with a new ambition to center family and community in our lives, moving away from the sterile habit of economic production and wealth accumulation. That would indeed be transformative.

From Crisis to Opportunity: Rethinking Education in the Wake of COVID-19

Connie Bird and Hidesh Bhardwaj

When the coronavirus disease of 2019 (COVID-19) outbreak began, it seemed to advance overnight and turn our world upside down without warning. The crisis has caused us to change almost every aspect of our lives – closing businesses, limiting interaction, and even canceling in-school classes for all K-12 students. There is no doubt that dealing with this global pandemic has been difficult for most people, but like all other crises, the challenges created by COVID-19 offer opportunities to build resilience, think creatively to solve problems, and emerge in a better place.

When classes in Alberta, Canada were canceled on March 15, thousands of educators around the province were immediately vacuumed into a whirlwind of figuring out how to ensure students would continue to learn. In a short time, remote learning systems were created and made available for students. Although the systems created in crisis response are a far cry from healthy, remote learning situations, the lessons we learn from this experience have the potential to power an evolution in education.

With the urgency and many challenges of moving to new ways of teaching and learning, educators have shown themselves to be a creative and responsive group of professionals. While making the quick transition to primarily online learning, many teachers have learned to use new online tools and platforms, created new ways of delivering lessons and working with students, and shifted their focus in assessment away from an evaluative process to one centered on improving student learning. While some teachers are attempting (and struggling) to move their old practices into an online arena, many are taking advantage of this unique opportunity to implement innovative changes. One strategy that is showing promise in supporting a greater number of students is recording and posting lessons online, allowing students to view lessons as many times as they need on their own schedule. When students are able to work at their own pace, it alleviates the pressure of keeping up to their peers. This offers students the time and space to connect, reflect, and create questions and ideas to help them develop deeper understanding. The time teachers save giving live lessons to entire classes can be used to work with students in small groups or one on one to provide more personal, timely feedback and support.

Another action some teachers are taking is to learn about and use different web-based learning programs, specifically for numeracy and literacy. In addition to saving time and providing independent practice, the benefit to many of these educational programs is their ability to identify learning levels for students and provide activities that are appropriately challenging to optimize learning. The analytics built into many programs bring another benefit – teachers are informed in real time of what their students are doing well and more importantly, where they need support, creating opportunities to further personalize learning for students.

These tools and strategies, along with several more, have helped meet the range of socio-emotional, academic, and scheduling needs of more students. As a result, many students who struggled in school are showing drastic improvements. Students with anxiety are more comfortable working alone from their own space. Students with attention challenges are having success working on their own schedule. Students who display challenging behavior in the classroom are not in conflict with their teachers, allowing for a more positive experience and more time engaged in learning. Many of these strategies are used in alternative settings however they are proving to be effective with numerous students in the mainstream as well. Educators are learning that the strategies and tools being used to get through this crisis can actually support teachers to personalize learning, engage more students and increase their connection with students. It would seem that many so-called 'alternative' approaches are actually beneficial for more of our students that we thought.

While it is clear that COVID-19 has created an opportunity to increase the breadth and depth of understanding of alternatives to classroom-based learning. The movement towards non-classroom based learning was captured by the Fraser Institute (2017) who reported that 9 of 10 provinces in Canada saw an increase in homeschooling enrollment between the 2007/08 and 2014/15 school years. This, paralleled the expansion of online high school programs and developments in brain sciencewhich have long since highlighted the desire and need for us to reimagine education and provide alternatives to classroom-based learning. The crisis created by COVID-19 has made evident the endless possibilities. Additionally, the impact of school closures has gone beyond individual students and teachers. From families to policy makers, all have witnessed the system's capacity to respond and adjust to the needs of students in a time of crisis; a shift that might have previously been seen as impossible. From this increased knowledge and experience comes new hope for those students who have previously floundered, or even chose to be absent from the mainstream public education system. Particularly for those children and youth exposed to histories of abuse or intergenerational trauma, these new opportunities might be the answer they have been waiting for.

Whenever school communities return to their school buildings and begin to heal and recover from this trauma, it is crucial that we bring the lessons learned during COVID-19 back to our school communities. With everything we are experiencing, it would be irresponsible to fall back to pre-COVID-19 education practice. The strategies and tools we are learning to use can help transform our schools into flexible hubs that use a variety of methods and strategies to meet the needs of all students.

Reference

Fraser Institute. (2017). *Homeschooling in Canada continues to grow*

The Distressing Levels of the Covid-19 Crisis

Jess Boon

I am a professional community counselor in Vancouver working within the field of social work, and for 10 years I have predominantly worked with youth in the foster care system and those who have aged out. As such, I offer this commentary and some concerns about youth work in the time of this pandemic. Like many people in my community, I respect and thank our front-line health care workers who work long shifts every day, treating patients during the crisis.

In Vancouver, where I live, many people have already been experiencing a fragile state for some time. For the past decade the city has notoriously suffered a housing affordability crisis at the same time as a contaminated opioid overdose epidemic which continues to claims thousands of lives every year. Recent Coroner's Service data suggest the deaths from that epidemic have accelerated during Covid-19. The extreme costs of living in British Columbia's Lower Mainland, and the vicarious community trauma caused by normalizing years of overdose deaths and suffering has made an already moody city of Vancouver even moodier.

I am a moody Vancouverite through and through, and I know that this city has been nervously standing on fragile glass floors for many years. I know even that many of the people around me who say they are doing "ok" are often hiding behind their pride and are in reality just scraping by cheque-to-cheque.

Overall, my immediate and future concerns for families and communities fall under three themes. I am most concerned about trends around job and economic security, the impact of the pandemic on children and youth, and mental health and isolation of vulnerable communities.

Jobs and economic security

I am concerned about the overall economic and job security of the people and how current government spending will impact the decisions of future administrations. The economy has been drastically impacted by the temporary closing and downsizing of businesses during Covid-19. Many middle class Canadian workers who had steady employment were forced to begin applying for government benefits for the first time in their lives after their industries suddenly shuttered.

It's important to know the scale of the issue. At this moment, the main social safety net for Canadians who have been laid off has been the Canadian Emergency Response Benefit (CERB).

According to statistics provided by the Statistics Canada (2020a, 2020b) as of June 4, 2020, 15.4 million CERB applications have been processed and $43.5 billion have been paid in benefits. We can only hope the CERB will be adequate to assist workers get back on their feet until it is safe to return to their workplaces post-Covid. We don't know yet what the long-term reality will be for workers.

Of course, I hope families impacted by the economic fallout of Covid-19 will recover their financial security, but considering record-high household debt in Canada even before the pandemic, I remain additionally concerned about an impending debt crisis that could last for years. I would not be surprised if during the pandemic more Canadians have been forced to rely on high-interest credit cards to pay for essentials, or resort to predatory payday loans to pay their rent, especially if they have been found ineligible for CERB or other benefits. Accessing high-interest credit and payday loans often becomes a ruthless cycle—and successfully overcoming debt becomes a real barrier in pursuing one's goals. When people have crushing debt, they often put off personal goals such as getting an education, ensuring stable housing, making long-term investments such as cars or houses, or starting a family. In other words, people get stuck.

I worry that these benefits, though needed, will result in cutbacks that could impact families in years ahead, if governments tighten their belts. Which services and budgets are going to get cut?

I am mostly bringing this up because I have my own selfish stake as an average millennial trudging through what feels like a dystopian societal nightmare that will impact everyone for decades to come. Throughout my life and career, all I have known is policies of austerity and, to be frank, it's just not been a good time.

Mental health

I am also concerned about the impending mental health crisis that seems absolutely inevitable. It doesn't matter who you are, humans are inherently social creatures and not built to spend this much time alone. When we are lonely, it's only a matter of time until past painful memories or thoughts begin to bubble to the surface and manifest. Even for those who were 'lucky' to be stuck within their homes with direct family or the truly introverted, people do usually draw supports from an extended community of coworkers and friends.

Also, before Covid-19, there were already so many people who were highly vulnerable in regards to community isolation. In my community of East Vancouver, many folks are seniors, living on disability benefits, experiencing homelessness and/or trauma-related addiction. Many of them were suddenly cut off from much-needed resources as many shelters, counseling services and non-profits were forced to close or reduce hours. I salute all the organizations that attempted to remain in touch with clients through virtual platforms, but truly there is nothing that can replace face-to-face interaction and supports. I am concerned that this pandemic will be the trigger event for many people who are already struggling with isolation and insecurity and that many will turn to self-medicating even more with substances, self-harming and/or dying by suicide.

Children and youth

Finally, I am concerned that young people may experience Covid-19 as a strange collective and even generational trauma. Children and youth growing up during this time are not only experiencing a pandemic but also processing it through the lens of hyper-technology and smart phones. Users of social media are often bombarded with emotionally charged content and information that is continuously consumed. I am an older millennial and I am worried about my younger peers who are considered to be a part of Gen Z. This is a generation of youth who are viewing both traumatic stories of Covid-19 cases and distressing images of police brutality against people of color. I know I can't take phones away from my younger peers, and I also know that ultimately there is importance in bearing witness to these images that show real human injustices. But I am genuinely concerned about ongoing consumption of such deeply traumatic images – ones that will likely impact the mental health, short- and long-term happiness, and overall well-being of the current youth generation. I also think it's important to listen to the voices of young activists who are currently participating on the front lines of the Black Lives Matter movement and, if asked, offer any tangible resources that might be needed during this time.

I am not even scratching the surface of the potential ramifications of Covid-19. However, I believe those working in our field should be mindful and begin ongoing conversations with colleagues about long-term trends in the economy, financial benefit programs, levels of Canadian household debt, and the mental health of both vulnerable communities and youth populations during and after Covid-19.

References

Statistics Canada. (2020a, June 10). *Stat-Can Covid-19: Data insights for a better Canada.* Retrieved June 21, 2020, from https://www150.statcan.gc.ca/n1/pub/45-28-0001/2020001/article/00030-eng.htm

Statistics Canada. (2020b, June 8). *Canadian emergency response statistics.* Retrieved June 21, 2020, from https://www.canada.ca/en/services/benefits/ei/claims-report.html

Building Resilience in Covid-19

Andrea V. Breen and Heather Chalmers

The impacts of COVID-19 on families in Canada are as diverse as the families themselves. There are family members navigating job demands while homeschooling, working in jobs that put them at heightened risk, and many who are now struggling to manage without a regular paycheck. There are families facing illness and others who are mourning loved ones. Some families are isolating together in comfortable homes with yards of their own while others are overcrowded with little or no access to the outdoors. For some, home may be a loving sanctuary and for others it may be a prison of conflict and violence. Most of us are missing people we love, and for families separated from loved ones in long term care homes, due to distance, or through involvement with the justice or child welfare systems, lock-down may be especially agonizing.

One commonality may be that in some ways, the clocks have slowed. In many families, meals are being prepared and eaten together, stories are being shared, art is being created, family connections are being strengthened, and families may have time to breathe. Many families are finding their ways to new routines, learning new ways to connect, and figuring out how to adjust their activities to prioritize well-being. For families who have time and access to the internet, this may be an opportunity to develop new skills. Exposure to culture and arts has become more accessible through virtual tours of museums around the world, art and music lessons, and virtual travel to places some may not have otherwise had an opportunity to visit.

Children and youth are finding ways to entertain themselves and stay connected with friends while in lock-down. There are drive-by birthday parades and creative group video gaming is becoming more heavily utilized. But for many, this time of isolation may be stoking the flames of new or preexisting mental health challenges. Loneliness, a lack of routine, and inadequate access to supports make this a dangerous time for many young people. Children and youth may feel that adults do not understand what they are going through and they are not wrong—none of us knows what it feels like to be 8 or 16 or 21 during a global pandemic. And many parents and caregivers are overburdened by their own worries to be able to give their kids the support they need.

Our kids are also experiencing additional disappointments. They are missing out on graduations and other celebrations that they may have spent years dreaming about. This fall, new postsecondary students will most likely be missing out on the typical first year experience. The economic crisis has led to job loss in all age brackets and this will hit postsecondary students hard. Students may need to postpone postsecondary studies and some who were planning to attend may no longer be able to afford it. Many young people are feeling uncertain and scared for the future. This pandemic will change the trajectory of the rest of their lives in ways that we cannot foresee.

While some parents and caregivers may be especially concerned about homeschooling and feeling pressured to keep up with formal learning, the really important lessons right now have to do with compassion and care, for ourselves and for each other. This may be a good time to reevaluate what is necessary. If the kids in our care are learning each day about how to help themselves feel just a little braver, more hopeful, and peaceful, then they are learning one of the most important lessons they can—they are learning to develop their own resilience in the face of adversity.

The entire world is facing the same crisis with COVID-19, and this highlights how we are truly all connected. While isolation has walled us off from each other in our separate family units, our ability to be resilient is not only dependent on our success in establishing healthy routines, learning new skills,and caring for our own loved ones. We think it is also about expanding our circle of care beyond our own families in safe and creative ways.

Coronavirus Challenges for Family Social Workers in Hong Kong

Simon Chan

This sharing is a reflection on the impact of COVID-19 on social work practices for children and families in Hong Kong. The implications for social work practices and education will also be discussed.

In December 2019, the first cases of COVID-19 emerged in Wuhan. Wuhan and other Hubei cities were subsequently placed under lockdown for nearly three months to contain the virus. Aside from Wuhan, Hong Kong was among the first group of Chinese cities that declared confirmed cases of COVID-19. Hong Kong was a British colony for 99 years until 1997 when its political administration was returned to China. Afterwards, Hong Kong has continued its role as a global financial center. However, even this cosmopolitan city cannot avoid the spread of coronavirus outbreaks. In 2003, the severe acute respiratory syndrome (SARS) appeared in Hong Kong and 1755 people became infected, which included some 360 hospital workers, who were initially unaware of the cause of the virus and took relatively few precautions. The community outbreak also led to the evacuation of infected residents to holiday camps. Ultimatey, 299 people died in Hong Kong in the spring of 2003, which is a fatality rate of 17 per cent. At the time, the SARS epidemic was considered the darkest period in the history of Hong Kong since its handover to China in 1997.

Little did Hong Kong and its residents know that the SARS epidemic would pale in comparison to COVID-19. The work and position of social workers in Hong Kong, especially those who provide services to children and families, would become greatly challenged in the face of this unprecedented pandemic. To gain a better sense of their experiences, seven social workers from children and family services, with working experience ranging from three to twelve years, were interviewed on how they continued to provide services, addressed the difficulties and challenges encountered, and finally, how they positioned themselves.

The seven social workers stated that COVID-19 has had negative impacts on children and families; in particular, explicit increases in incidents of family conflict and violence, and collective depression and panic among family and clan members, although fewer incidents of the latter were found when Hong Kong reported zero cases for more than two weeks in May 2020. On the other hand, unreported positive side effects were also found. For instance, the lockdown of the city gave self-isolating social service recipients and their family members the unexpected opportunity to spend more time together, which is a luxury in rapid paced Hong Kong.

In the face of the sudden changes demanded of children and family services, the social workers had difficulties in adjusting to the increases in family conflict cases including family violence, and mental health cases, including clients who began to experience depression. They were frustrated with the lack of capacity to manage their cases remotely. In fact, they themselves were also traumatized from the 'panicked' community response to COVID-19, such as empty shelves in the grocery shops, and shutting down of theaters and schools. Finally, they had to adjust to virtual means of contact instead of more personal and professional face to face meetings with their clients.

The social workers also reflected on their position during the process of adjusting to the new normal with COVID-19. They reflected on their role as a social worker for families with disadvantaged children and parents. During the past two months of lockdown in Hong Kong, most services for children and families have been limited and obviously no in-person office interviews or family visits have been provided, nor can there be manual applications made and submitted for resources. As such, the social workers questioned the value of social work in prioritizing the needs of clients; that is, how should the safety of social workers and immediate needs of clients be balanced in the face of COVID-19?

The social workers also reflected on their training and education with two lines of thought. While some felt helpless and frustrated about the shortcomings of the social work curriculum that has not prepared them for such a pandemic, others are reminded of the need to better equip themselves with knowledge on the use of online platforms in the long run. Nevertheless, there are two sides of a coin; sometimes challenges are also opportunities. Therefore, there is now the opportunity to expand social work to include more prevalent use of online education platforms, online casework and family services, and even online group sessions.

While the pandemic has both negative and positive ramifications for children and families, family conflict and family mental health issues are only the short-term effects. The sharing session delved into the role and position of social workers not only during this coronavirus but also the value of social work in Hong Kong. There will be other unforeseeable long-term negative and also positive impacts of the pandemic on the children and their families. That is the yet another challenge that social workers need to anticipate and prepare themselves for in order to fully meet the needs of their clienteles. Another crucial issue is how social workers should balance social work principles and values during such unprecedented times.

Last but not least, the social work curriculum and post-qualification training are concerns of these social workers. The deficiencies of their education as evidenced by the pandemic have been made alarmingly explicit. As such, how should the tertiary institutes in Hong Kong tailor their curriculum to address the challenges faced by children and their families in the 'new normal'? The professional body also has the responsibility to provide post-qualification training. More importantly is that the experience in Hong Kong as a bicultural city in dealing with COVID-19 can be used as a reference for other Mainland Chinese cities and/or provinces. Community and social workers in Mainland China have played an important role during this time in supporting disadvantaged children and families. Evidently, it is seen as an urgent task to determine how social service delivery should be enhanced in the long run to meet the needs of the children and families there. How Wuhan or other Chinese regions make use of the experience of Hong Kong is critical as they proceed toward their own 'new normal'.

Reflections on Being Oppression-Adjacent in the Time of COVID

David Collins and Jeremy Christopher Kohomban

We have personally been on the frontlines of the COVID-19 pandemic since early March, when it cascaded through our neighborhoods and upended our daily lives, and we have seen first-hand what is widely and correctly observed: the devastation of the pandemic both illuminates and exacerbates deep disparities in our society. Most notable among these are the wide gaps in wellbeing and opportunity on the basis of race, immigration status, class, neighborhood, and other factors. People of color, immigrants, poor people, and other marginalized groups have been hit hardest by the virus itself, as well as by its broader impacts.

Here, in New York City, which for the first few months was the US epicenter of the virus, the Tale of Two Cities (Kohomban, 2014) plays on. While many are social distancing and working from home, working-class people of color are most likely to be required to work in-person, often in positions that do not provide the luxury of social distance. Many continue to depend on subways and buses for transportation to essential front-line jobs, but are still compensated at non-essential wages (Kohomban & Collins, 2017). They go home to dense, intentionally segregated neighborhoods (Rothstein, 2020) with low-quality housing, high rates of intentionally concentrated pollution (Kilani, 2019), and a lack of convenient access to health care, groceries, and other necessary services. In fact, as the reality of COVID first spread through the city, many of these essential workers watched as those with time and money emptied out the stores of sanitizer, wipes and groceries, leaving little for them when their turn to purchase finally came (WCBS, 2020). All of these factors add up to one horrifying outcome: COVID is killing Black and Latino people at twice the rate of whites and Asians (Oppel, 2020).

When we talk to our colleagues in the charitable sector, the conversation frequently turns to the ways this current crisis lays bare structural inequities that have grown steadily worse with time. However, most of us have not seriously reflected on how charities exist within, and sometimes perpetuate, that same ecosystem. While we have acknowledged our role (Quinones et al., 2020) in the history of child welfare – which contributed to today's overrepresentation of poor people of color in foster care, jails and homeless shelters – it is tempting to place that responsibility in the past, and believe we have been reformed. We are still coming to grips with the fact that even today, we work in an oppression-adjacent industry.

When we describe ourselves as oppression-adjacent, we mean that a large portion of our programs today are made necessary by ongoing oppression, in the form of structural racism, segregation, poverty, disinvestment and social exclusion. They exist because the government has delegated much of the essential work of ensuring human wellbeing and opportunity to the charitable sector, which operates at lower cost and with greater precarity than the public safety nets that exist in most of the developed world and even in some emerging economies. And as these services have grown to fuel our institutions, in our advocacy we run the risk of substituting the interests of our institutions for the true needs and preferences of the people and communities we are privileged to serve.

In a just society, demand for some of our core services would be drastically reduced, and those that remain would look very different than they do now. If we do not have the courage to look toward that just world, and imagine its contours and details through our programs wherever possible, then we only prop up the oppression of today. Of course, imagination on its own is not enough. To the extent that the not-for-profit human services sector can serve as an innovation laboratory for government, providing proof of concept of new programs and approaches, we hope that these efforts may lead the government to adopt strategies that are more high-touch, community-driven, further upstream, less coercive and more focused on meeting the needs and preferences of those directly impacted.

There is nothing like a crisis to throw these dynamics into sharp focus. In our strategic plan here at The Children's Village, a child and youth-serving organization in New York City and its suburbs, we have reflected on our tendency to offer people what we have, rather than what they need. Nowhere is this more obvious than if we were to offer people the same old services – counseling, therapy and referrals – during a pandemic. Instead, over these last few months, we have pivoted to providing direct material aid to youth, families, foster families, and communities. This means not just money for food, clothing, or shelter, but access to smartphones, tablets, laptops and broadband internet, so families can stay connected and keep up with school. Private donors and foundations have stepped up to help meet this need, and our local government has also provided flexibility in the use of program funds for these purposes.

Though every social worker learns about Maslow's hierarchy of needs in their first week of classes, it is unfortunately not the norm in our profession to direct our resources first to the basic safety and health needs of our clients. This is because our dominant political and cultural values have always treated poverty (particularly amongst racialized peoples) as a moral failing and poor people as untrustworthy. The result has been the creation of strictly means-tested systems (Kohomban & Collins, 2017) that are more adept at surveillance and control than they are at providing aid. These attitudes have been absorbed by the local charitable sector and exported internationally as well (Doane, 2019). At times, in the child welfare system, we act as if the worst possible outcome is not for a child to be permanently separated from a loving family, but rather for some unworthy parent to get a little more help than they "deserve." If we did not see the harmfulness of this worldview before, we should all certainly be able to see it now.

The dangers of COVID have also forced our system in New York City to rethink standards and practices related to in-person contact with families. Unfortunately, for several months this meant that many children in foster care did not visit with family members, or did not see them as frequently. However, we did identify those children who could immediately return to their families and ride out the pandemic at home instead of in foster care. If material support was needed to help that family care for that child, we provided it. Caseworkers also received the flexibility to conduct many of their home visits by phone or video, rather than in-person.

For years, many advocates have argued that even child welfare services that are intended to be supportive, such as prevention or aftercare, often feel like surveillance to families. Now, we are finding that we can have more frequent, less intrusive, and more constructive interactions by using phone or video, rather than haggling over the timing of in-person visits, or forcing families to travel to our offices. We are able to start by asking if families have what they need; in this way, the concept of 'checking on their wellbeing' is needs-driven and controlled by the families rather than 'expert' social workers. Meanwhile, investigations and removals are down, and there has been no increase in serious safety issues among families who are remaining at home. Going forward, we should keep this more individualized approach to safety and supervision, and strive to have even more constructive and less coercive relationships with families.

We hope that we can keep the clarity of this moment, and the lessons it has provided, close at hand long after this pandemic is over. If we fail to do so, we will deserve every critique we receive as a result. Here are a few other ways we hope our sector and our city can change as a result of this crisis:

First, we must address the lack of safe, affordable, high quality, *integrated* housing in New York City. So much of the trauma and intergenerational disadvantage experienced by our families stems from this primary issue. In 2015, we partnered with Harlem Dowling to build nine stories of permanently affordable housing in the heart of Harlem, as proof of concept that affordability can be safe, beautiful, and accessible, filled with light and open spaces - just like those city dwellings enjoyed by the privileged.

But we will not solve this problem one building at a time. In *The Cities We Need* (New York Times Editorial Board, 2020), the editorial board of the New York Times observed how the engines of segregation, failing schools and unaffordability have combined to threaten our democracy and the promise of America's cities as engines of growth and innovation. There can be no permanent, high-quality affordable housing without integration – by race as well as by wealth. The people performing the work that makes New York City's neighborhoods so desirable – line cooks, child care workers, home health aides, artists, cab drivers, and many more – must be able to live here as well. Otherwise, those of us who remain are parasites, enjoying the culture and service of oppressed people without being willing to let them share in our opportunities. On this point, leaders in the charitable sector and their donors have rarely led by example. While a few give voice to the problem, most do not. Some simply don't care; others are afraid to offend their colleagues or funders, or are quietly happy with the status quo that allows them to avoid sharing their schools, neighborhoods and communities with the poor and people of color who serve them.

Second, we need to ask ourselves *before* we undertake any program or contract, whether it is structured in a way that helps make transformative change in peoples' lives. Our interventions should be designed to help people make lasting improvements in their health, wellbeing and quality of life, not just to apply a meager balm to the burning pain of intergenerational oppression. And we must respect the self-determination of the people served, by responding to their needs and preferences and including them in organizational decision-making processes. When we do continue to operate programs historically linked to family separation driven by poverty, explicit discrimination and oppression – such as residential schools or foster care programs – then we must work toward a near future where those programs are dramatically shrunk, transformed, or even eliminated. In the last thirty years, New York City has gone from having 50,000 children in foster care to less than 8,000. We believe that number can be reduced further still.

Finally, in that same vein of seeking to be sites of transformation and opportunity, we need to address the fact that our own organizations can be sites of oppression as employers, too. Not only are our clients mostly poor people of color, but in Human Services our workforce is heavily dependent on people (especially women) of color, and many of our jobs still pay poverty wages. In this sense, being oppression-adjacent is a double-edged sword; many of our programs exist because of intractable poverty and oppression in segregated neighborhoods, while many of our jobs fail to offer a path to prosperity for people from the very same communities. And while locally and internationally, our frontline workforce is predominantly black, brown, and female, many of us remain snowcapped (Schneiderman, 2019) – that is, disproportionately white (and male) at the top. This helps ensure that people of color remain locked in frontline jobs that expose them to higher risk from COVID-19, and indeed, from any health, financial or ecological crisis.

Addressing this situation requires a two-pronged approach as employers: first, we need to make sure that all front line jobs pay a living wage, so that people who do them can raise a family and enjoy a decent quality of life. Second, we need to create viable pathways to advancement for those faithfully serving on the frontlines at all levels of our organizations. You shouldn't have to be an executive to have a rewarding career in the charitable sector – but you shouldn't be prevented from working your way up if you want to, either. We must make sure that our leadership reflects and authentically represents frontline experience, the front-line workforce and the communities we serve. Finally, we must push for increased investment in our workforce alongside, and in tandem with, prioritizing the aforementioned need to channel more program resources directly to families and communities. Only then will we be able to offer transformative opportunities to our employees as well as our clients.

We don't put forward these recommendations to suggest that we have it all figured out. Like most dealing with this pandemic, we have struggled bravely together, and experienced our fair share of successes as well as mistakes. We have lost colleagues, family members and loved ones – because New York City has been at the epicenter of the crisis, and because our workforce is concentrated in its hardest-hit communities. Naming and describing the peculiar condition of being oppression-adjacent during a pandemic does not exempt us from critique. In fact, it requires us to accept that powerful institutions will always be critiqued by those who feel they have been excluded or mistreated. Despite being a historical charity founded in 1851, we do not feel powerful in the grand scheme of New York City politics – but we still exercise tremendous power over our clients and their communities. We have to accept those critiques and do better as we move forward, knowing that the edge of oppression is always a site of struggle and conflict.

The question becomes – if you are oppression-adjacent, which way will you push? We hope to always push toward a more just future, as best we can envision it.

References

Doane, D. (2019, December 10). Are INGOs ready to give up power? *OpenDemocracy.Org*. https://www.opendemocracy.net/en/transformation/are-ingos-ready-give-power/

Kilani, H. (2019, April 4). "Asthma alley": Why minorities bear burden of pollution inequity caused by white people. *The Guardian*. https://www.theguardian.com/us-news/2019/apr/04/new-york-south-bronx-minorities-pollution-inequity

Kohomban, J. C., & Collins, D. (2017, February 24). The systematic starvation of those who do good (SSIR). *Stanford Social Innovation Review*. https://ssir.org/articles/entry/the_systematic_starvation_of_those_who_do_good

Kohomban, J. C. (2014, March 8). New York the tale of two cities. *Huffington Post*. https://www.huffpost.com/entry/new-york-the-tale-of-two-_b_4548556?utm_hp_ref=tw

Oppel, R. A. (2020, July 10). *The fullest look yet at the racial inequity of coronavirus*. https://www.nytimes.com/interactive/2020/07/05/us/coronavirus-latinos-african-americans-cdc-data.html

Quinones, K., Kohomban, J. C., Collins, D. (2020, January 1). *Children's Bureau express*. US Department of Health and Human Services Administration for Children and Families. https://cbexpress.acf.hhs.gov/index.cfm?event=website.viewArticles&issueid=212§ionid=2&articleid=5479

Rothstein, R. (2020, January 20). The neighborhoods we will not share. *New York Times*. https://www.nytimes.com/2020/01/20/opinion/fair-housing-act-trump.html

Schneiderman, J. (2019, September 17). Nonprofit Leadership at a Crossroads. *Non Profit News, Nonprofit Quarterly*. https://nonprofitquarterly.org/nonprofit-leadership-at-a-crossroads

The New York Times Editorial Board. (2020, May 11). The cities we need. *The New York Times*. https://www.nytimes.com/2020/05/11/opinion/sunday/coronavirus-us-cities-inequality.html

WCBS.880. (2020, March 13). *Panic buying: Shoppers throng NYC stores amid coronavirus fears*. https://Wcbs880.Radio.Com. https://wcbs880.radio.com/articles/throng-nyc-stores-amid-coronavirus-fears

Wikipedia contributors. (2020, July 17). Maslow's hierarchy of needs. *Wikipedia*. https://en.wikipedia.org/wiki/Maslow%27s_hierarchy_of_needs

OPEN ACCESS

Social Protection: An Essential and Effective Social Policy Response During and After COVID-19

Julie L. Drolet

The global health pandemic due to COVID-19 has demonstrated the importance of expanding and adapting social protection measures. As the global spread of the virus moves from Europe, North America and East Asia to increasingly lower middle income and lower income countries, now is the time for innovation to support the health and well-being of people. With several billion people in lockdowns to enforce social distancing, social policy responses have emerged to address the socio-economic, health and environmental impacts.

The impacts of this pandemic are felt differently by different groups of people. Racialized and marginalized communities in America report worse health outcomes than other populations due, in part, to discriminatory practices in the health care system (CBC, 2020). The pandemic has revealed the interconnections and vulnerabilities between our social, economic, health and environment systems, and how working in public and private spaces impacts differently on different groups in the formal and informal economy. For example, who is classified as an essential worker providing essential services is a consideration in who can access personal protective equipment such as gowns, masks, gloves, and facial protection.

The 'Great Lockdown' is expected to have a devastating impact on the global economy that had already struggled with the collapse in world commodity prices. Social protection measures are essential to alleviate social and economic pressures experienced by the lockdowns. Workers in the informal economy often lack access to basic labor and social protections such as employment insurance, pensions, and related benefits (Drolet, 2016). The global pandemic has revealed the precarity of the lockdown measures on informal workers who have lost their livelihoods. This includes migrant workers, domestic workers, and home-based workers, among others.

The provision of essential health services and cash transfers has been widely adopted around the world to mitigate the risks and vulnerabilities affecting individuals and households from the shocks, stresses, and deprivations (Drolet, 2015). This is known as social protection. At a national level, social protection includes basic social security or social assistance guarantees aimed at preventing or alleviating poverty, vulnerability, social exclusion, and inequality (Drolet, 2014). This includes cash transfers and in-kind benefits such as income support benefits, pensions, and employment benefits, among others. This also includes economic assistance packages, tax moratoriums, social security contributions, wage subsidies, loans and guarantees for workers, and other benefits to increase access to health services, expand social services, and other in-kind supports.

COVID-19 has affected the lives of children and their families. With the closing of schools to prevent the spread of COVID-19, equal access to education and learning has emerged as a concern. Home-learning options with access to internet, books and schools supplies may not be available for all children. Children and youth are affected by their household's struggle to maintain livelihoods and income. Social protection through cash transfers, support for food and nutrition, and health services can mitigate the harsh impacts of the COVID-19 outbreak and response, particularly for children, youth and families in poverty.

In South Africa, social protection measures are providing relief to vulnerable households through social grants that were increased as of April 1, 2020 for older persons, war veterans, child grants, and care dependency grants (COVID-19 South African Online Portal, 2020). The government declared a national state of disaster and adopted containment measures, including social distancing, travel bans, screening at ports of entry, school closures, screening visits to homes, and introduced mobile technology to track and trace contacts of those infected.

Social protection coverage has grown exponentially in lower and middle-income countries in the decade following the 2008 financial crisis (Drolet, 2016). As is the case in South Africa and other countries, existing cash transfers can be scaled-up to alleviate financial barriers of families and households. However, additional measures beyond cash transfers can be adopted through support to frontline service providers and practitioners, access to health care, social services, flexible work arrangements, affordable childcare, and all governments should consider rapidly increasing coverage in response to the crisis and planning for continued social protection measures in the long-term. Social protection initiatives such as the provision of food parcels for vulnerable individuals and households, a measure recently announced by the Kingdom of the Government of Eswatini and in England, can get assistance into the hands of those who need it most.

Social protection is widely used as an effective instrument to reduce poverty, promote development, and increase resilience to shocks. Social protection has been used in disaster response, as 'a bridge between humanitarian assistance and development processes' (European Commission, 2019, p. 4) Social protection initiatives in times of disaster and humanitarian crises help to address the economic and social disruption that threatens the well-being of individuals, families, communities, and societies. It is critical that governments consider how to foster inclusion in social protection systems, while supporting livelihood recovery and the most vulnerable.

The ILO has urged governments to extend social protection to all and is advising on measures to promote employment retention, short-time work, paid leave and other subsidies, to ensure that economies, labor markets and industries will become stronger, more resilient and more sustainable when the pandemic resides (ILO, 2020).

Research is needed to collect data on innovative approaches to better understand the social and economic impacts of different measures to curb the spread of the pandemic. It is also important to consider the long-term impact and evaluation of measures taken by governments using different methods including social protection. While emergency social safety nets are critical during the pandemic crisis, it is imperative that governments plan for long-term measures to facilitate recovery and policies to achieve greater income security in the months and years ahead.

References

Bank of Canada. (2020). *COVID-19: Actions to support the economy and financial system.* https://www.bankofcanada.ca/markets/market-operations-liquidity-provision/covid-19-actions-support-economy-financial-system/

CBC (2020, 11 April). *As some states see black Americans hit harder by COVID-19, researchers call for detailed Canadian data.* https://www.cbc.ca/radio/thecurrent/the-current-for-april-9-2020-1.5527551/as-some-states-see-black-americans-hit-harder-by-covid-19-researchers-call-for-detailed-canadian-data-1.5528574

COVID-19 South African Online Portal. (2020). *Guidelines and relief – Social grants.* https://sacoronavirus.co.za/?__cf_chl_jschl_tk__=a8c9a642b1ac6703ee649fbd94cbd39c9a8af22c-1588100031-0-ATgs9VTvno5uYurdsRAeETvCD5r88Bl5_HJgdPvoMq3l-K8Y2PaVXmXCy1oAOOhZCw79xsQYt3XYZLhD0Rd3UqwEVT-TA2IkYynyP6WVZqk_DDR_gZfgCXy_SNH8yfhCWeYAfuobuMUNYV4SIxvEHrP174oZxeUm-HSm4QXK4sH3nRhgadr5R8WIkkaKAHoDAXFHeJ3tmYPOrxFMi3HP24Q5LgMs_fNvQxUr3s-u8JyiHc4zr4HOzhVgtpgrAgmlHvoQe3v-1KQPX7_gq4RNKuE

Drolet, J. (2014). *Social protection and social development: International initiatives.* Springer.

Drolet, J. (2015). Social protection: An alternative or not for Africa's post-2015 development agenda. In N. Andrews, E. N. Khalema, & N. T. Assié-Lumumba (Eds.) *Millennium development goals (MDGs) in retrospect: Africa's development beyond* (pp. 295–308). Springer.

Drolet, J. (Ed.) (2016). *Social work and social development perspectives on social protection.* Routledge.

European Commission. (2019). *Case study: Ethiopia.* Retrieved from https://europa.eu/capacity4dev/sp-nexus/documents/span-2019-case-study-ethiopia

ILO. (2020, 21 April). *COVID-19: How social and economic sectors are responding.* Retrieved April 22, 2020, from https://www.ilo.org/global/about-the-ilo/newsroom/news/WCMS_742203/lang–en/index.htm

The Immanence of Change: Who Will Write the History of COVID-19?

Kiaras Gharabaghi

All history is political. Whose history of COVID-19 is centered in the future also determines which politics are centered for the future. And it is by no means clear whose history will be centered, but it is likely that it will be a privileged history, written by privileged people, living in privileged places. In this way, nothing really will have changed; COVID-19 will not be a transformative catalyst for the ways we are together as communities or as societies, or even as a human race.

All politics are historical. The politics of any given moment is formed in the political patterns of the preceding moments, including the relations of power and voice. Ruptures in political history happen but only very rarely, and almost never for the good. The continuity of politics is maintained through exceptionalism. When the power of the day realizes the intelligence of the arguments for change and the necessity of transformation, it narrates these as exceptional, as outliers, as unusual. Evidence becomes contextual and contingent. This narrative states that climate disasters are tragic but there is no need to change the fundamentals contributing to climate change, because disasters are time limited. Wars are terrible, but no need to stop arming the warring factions, because wars are caused by exceptionally bad people. Whatever impulse for something new might appear, it is reduced to exceptional status such that the history of the moment is protected, and thereby its politics.

The most worrisome element of the current crisis is the rise of the new hero; frontline workers, grocery store clerks, and health care workers. We have declared them as heroes because their work, unfolding at great risk to themselves, keeps people alive. For decades, individuals have provided services in extremely adverse conditions, while people were dying, at great risk to themselves, but we did not declare them to be heroes. The Elder in an Indigenous community, whose wisdom and presence has kept that community alive, has never been declared a hero. The young woman caring for the families in the nearby tents in the Haitian refugee camp, in spite of the daily threat of rape and violence, was never declared a hero in spite of her work keeping people alive. The journalists and the intellectuals who risk their lives by speaking truth against the powers of the corrupt state are not declared as heroes although their words and their actions keep communities and their dreams alive. It seems only fitting that our new heroes are recognized for their sacrifices although this recognition comes with a politics that is anything but neutral, anything but celebratory, anything but innocent. Our new heroes are declared as such in order to be forgotten. Their heroism is contextual and contingent. In the absence of the pandemic, they will continue to do exactly the same things they are doing now but they will no longer be heroes. Just like dead soldiers, brought home from the war, celebrated as heroes on the way to their funeral. Post-celebration, they are not heroes – but they are still dead. During this pandemic, tens of thousands of 'heroes' have died; most of us cannot name even one of these heroes; instead, we move on to those who are still being heroes right now, still alive, not yet dead. And at some point, we realize the ugly truth of it all: it is not the individuals serving under these adverse conditions who we declare heroic; it is their contribution to allowing us to do nothing that is heroic. In fact, we are the heroes for doing nothing and surviving. We are the heroes for readying ourselves to go back to how things were not so long ago. Once the pandemic is over, we will celebrate ourselves and carry on with our entitlements.

Still, something will be different. A new shame, a new guilt will have emerged. We will not be able to deny our shameful treatment and abandonment of our elders; we will be conscious of the things we did not do to reach out to those less able to survive; we will know that this pandemic is not the end; it is a warning that our ways of being in this world are always at risk. And we will know that the next time, we may not survive, or at least a return to what we have come to expect from our ways of being in this world may not be possible.

The psychology of what comes next renders transformative change in how we are together immanent; that immanence, however, is contained by the history we will endorse, and by the politics we now allow. What will this history be? And what politics are we allowing?

There is nothing new in the formal politics of the day; these are now, as they have always been, characterized by the politics of latent blame. But there is something new in the informal politics of the day. The concept of care has risen again, and just for once, it has not been reduced to the patronizing ways of masculinity in our societies. Care, including the capacity to provide it using technical skills, and the courage to provide it using strength and confidence, is suddenly much more than a personal, or interpersonal act; it is sustenance for society, a prerequisite for economic survival, and indeed, a political force to be reckoned with. The uniform of care overshadows the military esthetic; personal protective equipment, complete with shields, gloves and masks, draws a rugged figure, a 'tough bastard', a relentless source of hope and actual survival. Just like the violence embedded in the military esthetic, the esthetic of care embeds power over life and death; as such, care is a form of violence, and violence always moves to the top of political, cultural and social narratives.

So, what does it all mean for young people, their families and their communities? The hope for the future rests on the transcendence of care through the spectrum from love to death; child care, youth care work, health care – these are the weapons deployed in 'the war against an invisible enemy'. Weaponizing care may not be what we thought a more humane future to entail; but it makes for a transformative history, and therefore a transformative politics. Those who provide care now are not heroes and should resist that label; they are the foot soldiers of immanence in the current moment. Care is violence of a higher order – it is the violence of love, dignity and community. If we can write the history of care, including the history of the wounded and the dead, we can move from immanence to revolution.

During a Pandemic, the Digital Divide, Racism and Social Class Collide: The Implications of COVID-19 for Black Students in High Schools

Sabrin Hassan and Beverly-Jean Daniel

A new strain of coronavirus, COVID-19, has emerged and has since caused the indefinite physical closure of schools in Ontario. Classroom instructions have moved to online platforms. The change to online schooling, though necessary, can be a significant barrier to accessing educational content for students who do not have full access to the Internet and technologies such as computers, laptops and iPads. Although there is no current data that speaks to technology access for Black students in Canada, one might extrapolate from longstanding trends in data pursuant to structural inequities impacting disproportionally Black and other racialized minorities that there may in fact be a digital and technological divide specifically impacting Black students negatively (Chakraborty & Bosman, 2005; Fairlie, 2004). Black students and their families are, as a result of systemic racism, overrepresented amongst precarious workers (Liu, 2019). They are often in unstable employment situations that include limited benefits. Frequently, they are faced with financial challenges that are exacerbated during this pandemic. They are also more likely to fall victim to the virus itself since the groups that are presenting with higher rates of COVID-19 infections, are more likely to live in precarious housing, fall within a lowered-income status, and be identified as immigrants and visible minorities (Wallace, 2020). In combination, these factors significantly increases the likelihood that some Black students' access to the required technologies is significantly compromised.

This limited access to technologies, can negatively impact Black students' educational growth and development and reduce levels of support from teachers and other school based staff such as child and youth care practitioners, social workers, and psychologist who all have the potential to play significant roles in their lives. Having limited access to consistent support systems that include the aforementioned school based staff can hinder promoting and building psychosocial factors that contribute to excelling academically, such as self-perception, attitudes, and intrinsic motivation (Codjoe, 2006). All of these factors can also impact the sense of community and/or connectedness, which can have implications for the mental health of Black students (Codjoe, 2006). Given the extent to which families are restricted to their homes, COVID-19 has the potential to lead to heightened anxiety levels and marginalization, further contributing to likely challenges in their schooling. What will all this mean for Black students in high school who are already subjected to systemic racism in their day-to-day lives and how will it be addressed when they return to school?

Given that Black students are at higher risk for dropping out of high school (Bajwa, et al., 2018; Codjoe, 2007; Collins & Magnan, 2018; Frenette, 2007; James & Brathwaite, 1996; Lennon, 2006) and have reduced rates of application to post-secondary institutions James and Turner (2017), this pandemic has the potential to even more significantly derail the academic pursuits of Black students, thereby generating lifelong impacts on the academic and career pathways of Black students, their families and the broader community. There are several factors that are colliding all at once and exacerbate an already tenuous reality for Black students. The interruption of their schooling, the lack of available of specialized or community-based supports, the misinformation and limited knowledge about this global pandemic, the experience of racism, combined with the inevitable challenges of adolescent development, presents an almost insurmountable challenge for many Black students to navigate. Implementing systemic responses now to address their needs for digital, technological, education and mental health supports are critical and time sensitive. This can ensure that Black students do not fall through cracks at a highly critical juncture in their academic journey

As has been the case in many social and institution systems, the lack of race-based data may be hiding deep structural issues that will impact disproportionally on Black students many years, perhaps even generations, to come. It is there imperative that a component of the implementation of a systemic response include the collection of disaggregated race-based data in order to address gaps in knowledge and support efforts in securing funding that can make fundamental change (Sinai Health System, n.d).

Equipped with real time data that a specifically illuminates the circumstances, material context and social consequences of inequities in education, housing, employment, technology and other contexts, a systemic and systematic response plan can be developed and implemented to ensure that Black students are supported, both now as the pandemic is still active, but also later, when an already problematic education system seeks to resume its operations. The specific needs of Black students must be taken into account to ensure they reach their potential academically and to ensure their overall mental and physical wellbeing.

References

Bajwa, J. K., Abai, M., Kidd, S., Couto, S., Akbari-Dibavar, A., & McKenzie, K. (2018). Examining the intersection of race, gender, class, and age on post-secondary education and career trajectories of refugees. *Refuge*, *34*(2), 113–123. https://doi.org/10.7202/1055582ar

Chakraborty, J., & Bosman, M. M. (2005). Measuring the digital divide in the United States: Race, income, and personal computer ownership. *The Professional Geographer*, *57*(3), 395–410. https://doi.org/10.1111/j.0033-0124.2005.00486.x

Codjoe, H. M. (2006). The role of an affirmed black cultural identity and heritage in the academic achievement of African-Canadian students. *Intercultural Education*, *17*(1), 33–54. https://doi.org/10.1080/14675980500502271

Codjoe, H. M. (2007). The importance of home environment and parental encouragement in the academic achievement of African-Canadian Youth. *Canadian Journal of Education / Revue Canadienne de L'éducation*, *30*(1), 137–156. https://doi.org/10.2307/20466629

Collins, T., & Magnan, M. (2018). Post-secondary pathways among second-generation immigrant youth of Haitian origin in Quebec. *Canadian Journal of Education*, *41*(2), 413–440.

Fairlie, R. W. (2004). Race and the digital divide. *Journal of Economic Analysis & Policy, De Gruyter*, *3*(1), 1–40. https://doi.org/10.2202/1538-0645.1263

Frenette, M. (2007). *Why are youth from lower income families less likely to attend university? Evidence from academic abilities, parental influences, and financial constraints. (Analytical Studies Branch Research Paper Series)*. Statistics Canada.

James, C. E., & Brathwaite, K. (1996). The education of African Canadians: Issues, contexts, and expectations. In K. Brathwaite & C. E. James (Eds.), *Educating African Canadians* (pp. 13–31). James Lorimer & Company Ltd.

James, C. E., & Turner, T. (2017). *Towards race equity in education: The schooling of black students in the Greater Toronto area*. York University.

Lennon, K. M. (2006). *A critical examination of academic success among black high school students in Toronto* (Order No. MR16227) (ProQuest Dissertations & Thesis A&I). ProQuest Dissertations & Theses Global. (304930868).

Liu, J. (2019). The precarious nature of work in the context of Canadian immigration: An intersectional analysis. *Canadian Ethnic Studies*, *51*(2), 169–185. https://doi.org/10.1353/ces.2019.0013

Sinai Health System. (n.d). *Black experiences in health care: Symposium report*. https://www.mountsinai.on.ca/about_us/human-rights/pdfs/SHS-BEHC- report-FINAL-aoda-final.pdf

Wallace, K. (2020, May 12). Toronto scientist dug into the connection between race, income, housing and COVID-19. What they found was 'alarming'. *The Star*. https://www.thestar.com/news/gta/2020/05/12/toronto-scientists-dug-into-the-connection-between-race-income-housing-and-covid-19-what-they-found-was-alarming.html

Hiding and Being Found: How Inequity Found Its Spotlight during COVID-19 and What It Means for the Future

Joy Henderson

At the time of writing this article, I have been in self isolation for seven or eight weeks, with three children and my partner, who is a Child and Youth Care practitioner. Like many, we are balancing staying safe, taking care of our family members, doing what little work we can do from home, finding ways to keep the anxiety in check and unsuccessfully preventing three brothers confined for too long from inventing new ways of annoying each other.

I was approached by the editors to describe what I think the positive or negative impacts of COVID-19 will be on young people. My most authentic response is "Hell if I know". Because I truly don't, nor can I imagine the impacts of long or short-term social isolation. I have no frame of reference for such an event. I don't even have the decades of studying theories to reference, so I am left to my experiences, cultural frameworks and a little bit of professional and personal instinct.

What I do know is how much COVID-19 has placed inequity under a giant spotlight. Whilst executives and celebrities self-isolate in their million dollar homes, thousands of workers deemed essential to keep us healthy, fed and entertained (somewhat) march off to work. What isn't lost on me is how many of these workers are women and/or racialized and paid minimum wage. Many Personal Support Workers (PSWs) work with dying senior populations in overcrowded long-term facilities without the proper protective gear and, as a result, become ill and sometimes die. We look at the US where states that collect race based health data illustrates that many who are dying are Black or Indigenous. Doctors without Borders (Crump, 2020) are flying into Navajo Nation (Navajo Nation, Department Water Resources, 2020) to deal with the highest amount of COVID19 cases per capita, whilst more than 30% of homes do not have access to running water. Meanwhile, my own province of Ontario, has finally agreed to collect race-based data after intense pressure from activists and political parties. The premise is that identifying race-based inequities will result in action, but activists are also realists and understand that action will only be taken after many hard conversations and organizing.

Youth from marginalized communities may have seen themselves become the primary income earner, if they have been deemed 'essential', they may have had to step up to become the caregiver whilst adults in their homes work multiple shifts to secure their jobs in times of precarious labor. Many youth are now faced with the realities of 'emergency remote learning', which governments are pushing through, not heeding the calls of equity- minded educators bringing up the myriad factors that make this learning inaccessible for many students, due to limited broadband, a lack of hardware, learning styles, or simply not enough devices in the home to cover young people as governments and privileged parents demand synchronous learning. Many CYCs are challenged with a lack of connection, virtual or otherwise, with our young people, because we rely heavily on publicly funded spaces to do our work with the young people who need it the most.

Meanwhile, we are horrified by reports of race-based killings of Black and Indigenous people such as Ahmaud Arbery, Eishia Hudson, Sean Reed, Breonna Taylor, George Floyd, Regis Korchinski Paquet, Chantel Moore, Jake Samson and Morris Cardinal. Black and Indigenous lives taken from this world because white supremacy has deemed jogging, hunting, or simply being at home to be criminal actions arbitrarily punished by death, either by the state or self-appointed arbitrators of state law.

What I am getting at with all of this is that in addition to the strange and unprecedented times where a handshake may result in death, young people who are racially marginalized are witnessing many ways in which their lives are considered 'lesser than' by the systems that govern us. And what they may not have is the support, the language or the guidance to work through this at home, and very few outlets for these important discussions to be had when we return to 'normal' life.

Desmond Cole (2019) recently published *The Skin, We're In*, which highlights the brutality of racism in Canada. Using police interactions, public education, community action and learning, he paints a picture that challenges Canadians to see that racism is very much alive and well in our society, and thus I would like to take this moment to remind Child and Youth Care that we too are not immune from this be that by outright direct harm in overt racist actions or the widespread refusal to identify and acknowledge a problem. We too must begin to examine this issue as many of us work with racially marginalized young people, who are coming not only from the trauma of social isolation and hyper-vigilance of avoiding a deadly virus, but the quiet and not so quiet messages they have received from our leaders that their lives and well beings do not hold the same value. That starts with hard conversations in CYC to begin examining our biases and complicity within our own ranks not addressing racism. Educators in Ontario have gathered expert in equity studies to have round-tables via Zoom, referred to as #4bigquestions. Weekly, they discuss the impact of racism on students within the education system. Participants watch the sessions and engage in conversations on social media and study groups. While this cannot replace the in person learning and meaningful discussions we must have, it is a COVID-19 response that can be under-taken by many whilst we remain at home.

I've seen many memes, tweets, commentaries about rebuilding the world so that we do not return to the normal that thrived off racism, poverty, misogyny, homophobia, ableism and the crushing of millions of people not considered ideal by white supremacy. I am aware of my privilege in writing this article, and that many who will be reading it may not necessarily be on the front line. They are academics, and writers, and managers, maybe some students, hopefully those who are in the position to start examining, challenging, destroying and rebuilding our own systems and philosophies not aligned with Eurocentric norms and frameworks built around white-ness. We have been complacent for far too long not pushing discussions around equity, not only around race, but gender, ability, sexual orientation and class. It has resulted in a status quo where too many young people 'fall through the cracks' and while governments and systems play a significant role in this, we too must take responsibility in that our field has been defined by Eurocentric norms and privileges and that results in a massive oversight of the most vulnerable. Perhaps this will help human service pro-fessionals understand how a racialized student struggling with remote learning isn't a matter of noncompliance, but a network of systems, (including our own) designed to keep students like them shut out.

COVID19 has illustrated brilliantly the lines already drawn in the proverb-ial sand for our racialized youth and if we are to be brutally honest about our practice, our work will need to evolve to having important conversations around equity for racially marginalized youth and practitioners. It is import-ant for us to use this time to make or strengthen our commitment to anti-racism work, pushing the tough conversations forward, and challenging our privilege and entrenched racism and most importantly, making room for workers and young people sharing their wisdom, knowledge and experiences.

References

Cole, D. (2019). *The skin we're in.* Anchor Canada.

Crump, J. (2020, May, 12). *Coronavirus: Doctors Without Borders sends Team to Navajo Nation, worst-hit area in the US.* The Independent UK.

Navajo Nation. (2020). *Department of Water Resources.* https://www.nndwr.navajo-nsn.gov/

COVID-19 Pandemic and Public Private Partnerships: Supporting Children and Young People

Sydney Henry

There is relevance to the perspective that we should 'never let a good crisis go to waste'. It could serve as the catalyst that brings out the best in us, pushing us to become better than we have ever been. And yet, this requires that we identify and trigger our latent human competencies - creating new experiences, new values and attitudes, new norms and a new culture.

This is true of the place of our children and youth in this COVID-19 crisis. They are half of the Jamaican population and more than half of the poor. Half of whom live in rural communities, half of whom have the distinction of being unattached and at risk and more than a half of whom are the victims and/or perpetrators of all serious crimes in the country.

As a student and practitioner of public policy and development studies, I am aware of the need to contribute to the present so as to ensure that those who will come after me will be able to enjoy as much as, or more than what I have had of the benefits to my existence. For this to happen, I must be able to interpret, reinterpret, understand and communicate the social construction of my own journey with academic rigor and passion in praxis.

Children and young people are a part of the development discourse but their place is determined by the purveyors of ideas whose configuration of outcomes are memes, hyperbole and clichéd rhetorical relationships. Our intervention of the Village Academy (School of Agriculture) is a social and institutional arrangement that recognizes the place of power in the social, economic and political construction of relationships that is able to define and determine sustainable change in the life experience of these young people. Our theory of change supports the disruption of the status quo and a redistribution of power, defined by purpose driven enterprise and innovation that is owned by young people. This ownership is situated in their knowledge, skills and aptitude to take responsibility for the rights that are inalienable to them as citizens.

It is and will be our youth who must be empowered to envision their local and global role in an international value chain that situates production not as a function of capital and equity, but of passion, cooperation and trust. These virtues are attracted to value-added innovations that are relevant to emergent needs of a people who are more cognizant of health and wellness and who value faith and family.

As a development practitioner, the purpose of my mission has been and continues to be, to cultivate relevant partners, whose mutual appreciation of profit is also of the determination of purpose in the lives of those marginalized and unattached children and youth. It is to create a living image of the new world of equals, dismissive of the utopian ideal of the end of poverty. One that is aggressive in the pursuit of the dignity of the human spirit and is empowered through self-determination and sustained through the character of community.

It is to negotiate and provide affordable access. Disruptive innovations of pathways to outcomes of success that are measured by wealth, the antithesis of being rich. Access on the scaffold of rights, roles and responsibility. That we would train young people through community based interventions, provide facilitators with global competence, expose them to the rigors of industry, the diversity of community and the collaboration of peers. Securing reliable resources that add value to the lives of young people should not only be seen as appendages or entitlements but rather as investments that will provide exponential returns for personal and collective good. Such approaches would not only support sustainability but also encourage young people to hold investors accountable. All this ought not to be an imposition upon our youth of a 'one size that fits all' but to support the reengineering of the reality from which they will have to make choices and own the process through which change will be experienced in their time and generation.

The COVID-19 pandemic has indeed provided opportunities for us to stop, think, refocus and prioritize. Investing in children and young people through partnerships with institutions sharing common goals remains center stage. Profit which reflect relevant partnerships, affordable access, passionate practitioners and reliable resources are the keys to change in the new dispensation, post COVID-19.

Covid-19 and Vulnerable Families Living in Rural Locations: Building a System for Recovery

Rochelle Hine, Andrea Reupert, Phillip Tchernegovski, Jade Sheen, and Darryl Maybery

Introduction

The COVID-19 pandemic has had profound implications for communities around the world. The physical health impacts of a pandemic alone are devastating, however the "mental health implications can last longer and have greater prevalence than the epidemic itself" (Ornell et al., 2020, p. 1). Common emotional responses to pandemics are similar to other catastrophic events such as war, and may include fear, anger, depression, anxiety and loneliness along with optimism and resilience (Smith et al., 2020). Many adults are reporting feeling overwhelmed, due to unemployment or loss of income, perceived threats to physical health and isolation (World Health Organisation, 2020). While an increased sense of solidarity ("we're all in this together"), has been reported, it is recognized that we are not all "in the same boat," and that socio-economic, gendered, cultural, racial and geographical disparities mean that the experience of COVID-19 will be more difficult for disadvantaged families who have fewer social and economic resources.

Children and families

The World Health Organisation Inter-Agency Standing Committee (IASC) Reference Group on Mental Health and Psychosocial Support in Emergency Settings (World Health Organisation, 2020) indicated that children require a protective environment encompassing active listening, increased care and sensitivity, opportunities to play and relax, regular routines and clear age-appropriate information regarding the pandemic. Unfortunately, carers' capacity to provide this environment may be compromised by their own biopsychosocial responses to the pandemic and its ramifications.

Rurality, risk and impacts

The majority of COVID-19 infections have occurred in urban settings. Previous pandemics show, however, that people do not need to be living in areas with high rates of infection to experience stress; sensational media reporting and the perception of risk are important factors in determining mental health (Blendon et al., 2004).

The closure of businesses, sporting clubs, schools, playgrounds, recreational spaces and social distancing laws prohibiting contact with family members, friends and neighbors have particularly affected rural communities. In rural locations, schools and sporting clubs play a critical role in providing community hubs and facilitating social connectedness. Physical distancing may be easier for those on farms or remote properties, however loneliness and isolation – always a risk for those in rural areas – may be experienced acutely (Repke & Ipsen, 2020).

Young people have identified access to education as a major concern during the pandemic (Youth Advisory Council of Victoria, 2020). Education is an important social determinant and a mechanism for overcoming transgenerational poverty and disadvantage (Reupert, 2020). The lockdown of schools has highlighted disparities between family groups. Some rural and disadvantaged families lack access to technology and have insufficient internet connectivity. Many families living with adversity may not have the skills, capacity and/or time to provide the stable, stimulating learning environment that can support their children's remote education, potentially perpetuating the cycle of disadvantage.

Stay at home requirements may feel more restrictive for Aboriginal families, where concepts of family and home are broad and can be more fluid (Gee et al., 2014). Aboriginal families can be comprised of members across households and generations. Being separated from aunts, uncles, grandparents and siblings may have a profound and detrimental impact for some children. Likewise, cultural and community sites may be conceptualized as an extension of home (Gee et al., 2014). Current restrictions may hamper cultural and spiritual activities, including connecting with and caring for Country.

Rural women already face increased risk of family violence due to a strong rural culture of masculinity, access to firearms and reduced service options (Campo & Tayton, 2015). This pandemic has seen an increase in family violence due to greater time spent at home under stressful circumstances including financial strain and increased alcohol consumption

(Clay & Parker, 2020). Children are at greater risk of being exposed to violence when home from school (Foster & Fletcher, 2020). If telephoning or telehealth are the only options for accessing support, some victims may not have an opportunity to safely make contact while the perpetrator is socially isolating or in quarantine with them.

Finally, some families are facing reduced access to food banks, community mental health, General Practitioners, dental services, family supports and sexual assault services. Rural hospitals that have limited capacity at the best of times have closed regular services to enable staff, infrastructure and resources to be diverted to COVID-19 responses.

Positive benefits

In response to COVID-19, telehealth, which has long been supported by evidence of positive experiences in some circumstances (Hawker et al., 1998; Yellowlees, 2016) has been vastly expanded into services that previously lacked experience. Comfort levels with utilizing such technology may increase with familiarity and a positive experience. Owen (2020) illustrated that if professionals and parents have the correct equipment, knowledge and training, telehealth "... is a viable alternative for some families, especially for those that would not be able to access F2F [face-to-face] counselling" (p. 47). They continue by recommending a "... a flexible hybrid mode of counselling, combining F2F with the convenience of VC [virtual communication]" (Owen, 2020 p. 47).

Moreover, benefits of quarantine may include the opportunity to spend more quality time at home with family. Stress relating to travel, social engagement and expectations may be reduced and parents and children may find more time for discovering pleasurable activities such as exercise, games, cooking and gardening.

Recovery beyond COVID-19

Access and equity must be our driving values when rebuilding communities, which many have argued the pre COVID-19 world did not provide. Rural communities are often portrayed as resilient through their experience of previous disasters such as bushfires, floods and drought; these experiences can inform recovery efforts (Ranscombe, 2020). Table 1 provides examples of how governments, schools and other organizations can deliver an integrated model of care to promote psychological and physical wellbeing for those who have been most negatively impacted by the pandemic and address existing barriers to access.

Table 1. Issues related to COVID-19 and post COVID-19 Actions for children and families.

Example issues	• Exposure to family violence • Significant parental experience of anxiety and/or depression with/without other preexisting major mental illness • Emotional, physical or sexual abuse and/or neglect • Extended periods of social isolation/sensory deprivation • Exposure to distressing news content without age appropriate explanations or discussions
Actions for government	• Increase funding for specialist family violence (FV), sexual assault (SA) and mental health (MH) sectors, and police specialist services. • Review new legislation with a gendered lens to determine impact on men and women. • Fund qualified allied health staff in all schools. • Ensure funding models include rural loading to account for distance and complexity. • Fund MH services to support children and parents. • Address workforce issues in child protection sector, increase funding and professional development. • Develop and disseminate resources to support adults to have age appropriate discussions with children about COVID-19. • Redress inequalities in internet access and prioritize rural areas for improvements.
Actions for schools and child, youth and family services	• Expand services to offer on-line and telehealth platforms in addition to face-to-face options. • Employ qualified allied health staff and resource wellbeing teams in all schools. • Facilitate peer support groups for vulnerable children and parents with mental illness with online options. • Implement trauma-informed care strategies in school and services. • Collaborate with Aboriginal or First Nations organizations to design culturally appropriate interventions that redress disadvantage in these populations. • Identify and redress environmental, institutional and attitudinal barriers to access for people with disabilities.
Actions for families and communities	• Promote help seeking behavior and open communication about FV, SA and mental illness. • Contact police to report DV incidents in neighborhoods. • Normalize emotional responses to COVID-19 utilizing evidence-based resources to prompt discussions with children and adults (e.g., British Psychological Society, 2020). • Ensure sporting clubs are gender inclusive and do not tolerate sexism, racism or homophobia. • Support churches to develop polices to prevent and report child abuse and family violence. • Include more reports from children's perspective in local newspapers and social media. • Check-in with vulnerable neighbors and family members. • Support small local businesses, including the arts.

References

Blendon, R. J., Benson, J. M., DesRoches, C. M., Raleigh, E., & Taylor-Clark, K. (2004). The public's response to severe acute respiratory syndrome in Toronto and the United States. *Clinical Infectious Diseases*, *38*(7), 925–931. https://doi.org/10.1086/382355

British Psychological Society (2020). *Advice for key worker parents: Helping your child adapt to changes due to COVID-19*. Retrieved May 14, 2020, from https://www.bps.org.uk/sites/www.bps.org.uk/files/Policy/Policy%20-%20Files/Advice%20for%20keyworker%20parents%20-%20helping%20your%20child%20adapt.pdf

Campo, M., Tayton, S. (2015). *Domestic and family violence in regional, rural and remote communities: An overview of key issues.* Retrieved May 05, 2020, from https://aifs.gov.au/cfca/publications/domestic-and-family-violence-regional-rural-and-remote-communities

Clay, J., & Parker, M. (2020). Alcohol use and misuse during the COVID-19 pandemic: A public health crisis? *The Lancet, 5* (5), 259. https://doi.org/10.1016/S2468-2667(20)30088-8

Foster, H., & Fletcher, A. (2020). *Women's Safety NSW update: Impacts on COVID-19 on Domestic and Family Violence in NSW.* Women's Safety NSW.

Gee, G., Dudgeon, P., Schultz, C., Hart, A., & Kelly, K. (2014). Aboriginal and Torres Strait Islander Social and Emotional Wellbeing. in Dudgeon, P., Milroy, H. & Walker, R., *Working Together: Aboriginal and Torres Strait Islander Mental Health and Wellbeing Principles and Practice.* Ch 4, pp 55–68.

Hawker, F., Kavanagh, S., Yellowlees, P., & Kalucy, R. (1998). Telepsychiatry in South Australia. *Journal of Telemedicine and Telecare, 4*(4), 187–194. https://doi.org/10.1258/1357633981932181

Ornell, F., Schuch, J., Sordi, A., & Kessler, F. (2020). "Pandemic fear" and COVID-19: mental health burden and strategies. *Brazilian Journal of Psychiatry, 42*(3), 232–235. https://doi.org/10.1590/1516-4446-2020-0008

Owen, N. (2020). Feasibility and acceptability of using telehealth for early intervention parent counselling. *Advances in Mental Health, 18*(1), 39–49. https://doi.org/10.1080/18387357.2019.1679026

Ranscombe, P. (2020). Rural areas at risk during COVID-19 pandemic. *The Lancet Infectious Diseases, 20*(5), 545. https://doi.org/10.1016/S1473-3099(20)30301-7

Repke, M., & Ipsen, C. (2020). Differences in social connectedness and perceived isolation among rural and urban adults with disabilities. *Disability and Health Journal, 13*(1), 100829. https://doi.org/10.1016/j.dhjo.2019.100829

Reupert, A. (2020). *Mental health and academic learning in schools: Approaches for facilitating the wellbeing of children and young people.* Routledge.

World Health Organisation. (2020). *Mental health and psychosocial considerations during The COVID-19 outbreak.* Retrieved May 05, 2020, from https://www.who.int/docs/default-source/coronaviruse/mental-health-considerations.pdf?sfvrsn=6d3578af_8

Yellowlees, P. (2016). Evidence for telemedicine in psychiatry. *Medscape Psychiatry*, 6th May. https://www.medscape.com/viewarticle/862604

Youth Advisory Council of Victoria. (2020). *COVID-19 and young people.* Retrieved May 06, 2020, from https://www.yacvic.org.au/assets/Documents/FINAL-Young-People-Survey-Results.pdf

COVID 19: The Precarity of Families and Disability

Rachelle Hole and Tim Stainton

Imagine you are home with your family during the covid-19 pandemic. You are limited to family only contact and minimal out of home activity. The kids are home schooling and you and your partner are trying to work from home. Money is tight and you cannot afford not to work. It's tough, but you cope, barely.

Now imagine that one of those children has a significant disability, is medically fragile and normally requires significant hours of support from workers to maintain their health and wellbeing and to allow you to work. Now you are trapped. The strain of trying to provide 24 hour care while trying to work and look after your other children takes its toll on you and your family. If and when workers are available you worry that they may bring the infection with them. Where have they been? Who have they been in contact with? PPE has not been made readily available adding to your concern.

The fear for the health of your child is palpable. They would not cope well with respiratory distress. If they get sick and need to be admitted to hospital, current visitation policy precludes visitors of any kind, despite the fact your child does not communicate through formal means and only those who know them well are able to interpret their communication. The thought of the sheer terror your child would experience while lying in a bed in a strange place with a room full of masked strangers is unbearable, so you resolve that unless it was clearly life or death you will not take your child to hospital. Even more frightening is the prospect that they might not even be treated as triage protocols may deem them low priority for scarce ventilators. You've seen that movie before when doctors, with looks of deep compassion, asked, "Do you really want them treated? We could just let them go; might be best for everyone."

You worry about your other children as well. They are forced to endure a more rigid lockdown due to fears of infection. They are also often last on the to do list after necessary care for your disabled child and work. All of this in a context of increasing tension within the household brought on by the stress and anxiety.

While COVID 19 is changing the world, it also has exposed the precarity of the vulnerable (i.e., persons with disabilities). Precarity is the "politically induced condition in which certain populations suffer from failing social and economic networks of support and become differentially exposed to injury, violence, and death" (Butler cited in McNeilly, 2015, p. 150). COVID 19 has uncovered systems that lack policies and practices to be responsive to the needs of individuals with disabilities (Lunsky et al., 2013). Moreover, these systems are frequently staffed by personnel without the awareness and knowledge to support and treat individuals with disabilities to produce equitable health outcomes within the confines of the current pandemic. This is more problematic when an underlying discourse permeates these policies and practices. That is, "What is a livable life?"

We engage with the concept of 'livability' as it incites critical questions about "which lives are viable and flourishing [and recognizes that] in particular socio-political contexts [this] is a fundamentally political activity, and one which, for Butler, holds possibilities to [realize] radical social transformation" (McNeilly, 2016). As such, how might we envision a society post-COVID 19 responsive to persons with disabilities and families where the socio-political context is positioned to support the livability of the children, youth and families in ways that see them thrive? What lessons do we take forward?

The Canadian Government has outlined their national response to COVID 19 for persons with disabilities [https://www.canada.ca/en/public-health/services/diseases/2019-novel-coronavirus-infection/guidance-documents/people-with-disabilities.html]. Outlined are suggestions for responding to the needs of disabled persons, health care advice and recognition of the particular needs of disabled persons and their families, such as the need for support persons to be allowed into health care facilities. What is absent is really any discussion of the needs of families in caring for their child or youth at home: recognition of the additional financial, emotional, and logistical challenges they face during public health emergencies such as the Covid-19 pandemic.

There has been significant progress made in recognizing that disabled people and their families face distinct challenges and require an intentional and focused response during public health crises. In Canada, nationally and in some provincial jurisdictions, we have seen government response groups formed to specifically consider the unique issues faced by disabled persons. That said, the needs of disabled youth, children and their families have received comparatively less attention. There must be recognition that the 'precarity of the vulnerable' discussed above is relational when it comes to children and youth with disabilities. That precarity ripples through the family system and must be addressed as such. So as we reflect on the lessons of Covid-19, we have learned much and made significant progress with regards to disabled persons, but there is much left to learn and disabled children, youth, and their families should be high on our collective list of areas where we need to do better.

ORCID

Rachelle Hole http://orcid.org/0000-0001-5238-0015

References

Lunsky Y., Klein-Geltink J. E., Yates E. A. (Eds.) (2013). *Atlas on the primary care of adults with developmental disabilities in Ontario*. Institute for Clinical Evaluative Sciences and Centre for Addiction and Mental Health.

McNeilly, K. (2015). From the right to life to the right to livability: Radically reapproaching 'life' in human rights politics. *Australian Feminist Law Journal*, *41*(1), 141–159. https://doi.org/10.1080/13200968.2015.1105771

McNeilly, K. (2016, May 26). *Livability: Notes on the thought of Judith Butler*. Retrieved May 25, 2020, from https://criticallegalthinking.com/2016/05/26/livability-judith-butler/

COVID-19 and Collective Grief

Shadan Hyder

The global pandemic has hurtled many of us into an unprecedented uncertainty in North America. For those of us who work the frontline, we may not have had the opportunity to process the tumultuous emotions that uncertainty brings, while simultaneously holding space for the emotions of others. Those we work under and for/with; employers, youth, families, are all sprinting to figure out how to provide support, while the majority of our traditional tools have been taken from us. The issues and barriers we were already dealing with have been exacerbated by a deadly virus and the makeshift adjustments of governments struggling to keep up. The burnout from working beyond our capacities with little to no pause, has taken us like a strong current, and it is hard to catch one's breath with the constant waves of 'new information', 'new COVID responses', 'new risks' and 'new deaths'. Here on the frontlines, it seems many of us are just trying to stay afloat.

Within the new parameters of a dangerous environment, and the ongoing exacerbation of existing systemic issues on marginalized peoples there is a nuanced grief and loss that people are experiencing- both tangible and intangible. Loss of freedom, people, structure, predictability, housing, food security, community, traditions, coping mechanisms, safety, physical touch… the list could go on. Given all of this, it can be assumed that we have been experiencing a collective grief and have been in mourning since quarantine has begun. Some of us are in our anger stage, some of us are still in denial, some bargaining, some depressed and some have begun acceptance of a new way of existing. These five stages are fluid, however, the ultimate and ideal goal for us to get to, and remain at, is the acceptance stage to begin life anew. For this new era, one in which pandemics probably will not be uncommon, I believe it is not just acceptance, but a radical acceptance that we must endeavor to reach. How does one come to this place? Radical acceptance entails not only wholly accepting life as it is, but to do so with an intentionality to grow and become stronger.

There are and always will be grief triggers around us, as we begin to slowly re-integrate into public spaces. The dire need to create new boundaries for safety purposes, as well as to support one's mental health during and after re-integration, are a large part of navigating this reintegration safely. No longer, at least not for a while, can one put a hand out and expect a hand shake in return. Ways of being and moving in social spaces need to be reimagined. Intimacy will need to be reimagined. A world reliant on social distancing or technological aids is not a world accessible to the majority. Harm reduction will need to be a large part of community spaces, spanning outside of its usual terrain. We will have to navigate our reliance on community care and support each other in doing so. Disability justice will need to be prioritized for those who are, and those who support, immuno-compromised people, in addition to racial justice to mitigate systemic barriers and impacts. We must look to our history and learn from past experiences of communal healing from collective grief.

From my personal observations, we can expect to continue to see responses to these new boundaries based on which stage of grief an individual is in. Some may be angry that others continue to socially distance. Some may believe that there is no longer a need to be concerned, and others may feel the need to justify why you can be near them. For many, accepting a new reality is difficult and sometimes painful as human nature makes us reluctant to isolate. Community is part of health, and we would be abject to deny it, despite health recommendations to keep apart. However, when one resists change, suffering is added to that pain, and elongates the distressful emotions experienced. To radically accept life as it is does not mean one is pliant when challenged, but rather demonstrates a person is in a place to assert themselves and stand steadfast in their boundaries, beliefs and values. All this while being able to accept how obscure life can be and the web of relationships within it. We must radically accept that we are all struggling and that is okay; that we are all going to be, for a while, in a perpetual state of 'okayness'.

This new era requires us to acknowledge the nuanced emotions of grief and loss we are experiencing and step forward into radical acceptance. Acceptance of having to ride the waves of grief and disruption without knowing what the waters hold but with perseverance to continue swimming, adapting to the currents, and creating tools from what is accessible to us. We must learn to be alright with floating in stillness when we need to, and we must be resilient in the midst of the numerous waves that seem to keep coming.

COVID-19 in the Era of Opioid Overdose: A Glimmer of Hope in the Midst of Double Whammy Tragedy

Mohamed Ibrahim

The global outbreak of the Corona virus has significantly impacted vulnerable individuals and communities across the world, including those who are homeless or precariously housed and dealing with addiction and complex health issues (British Columbia Center on Substance Use [BCCSU], 2020).

This reflective paper discusses the impact of COVID-19 for individuals and communities affected by the current opioid overdose crisis in British Columbians especially in the highly visible Downtown East Side (DTES) neighborhood of Vancouver which has been the focus since the COVID-19 regarding homelessness and overcrowding, and the potential devastating risk a COVID-19 outbreak. Although the short term outlook is bleak, the pandemic may actually lead to a more comprehensive harm reduction approach toward substance use and addiction in British Columbia and possibly in Canada.

On the 14th of April, 2016, the government of British Columbia declared opioid overdose as a public health emergency in response to the escalating mortalities from a poisoned street drugs supply chain with fentanyl, a deadly and highly potent synthetic opioid that is 100 times potent than heroin (NIDA, 2019). While there were about 200 deaths related to drug overdose in 2009 (BC Coroners Services, 2020), the death toll soared to1000 by 2016.

By declaring a public health emergency, the Act provides new set of powers to the Provincial Health Office (PHO) to ameliorate the social and health impact of the opioid pandemic at individual and community levels (BC Government, 2016). Those powers include implementing emergency measures, new regulations, and centralizing coordination and reporting across sectors. These measures focused at the individual level where free distribution of Naloxone; access to treatment; and encouraging drug users not to use alone since the majority of deaths are associated with individuals who used alone and died alone without any help. At the community level, measures focused on public health promotion and prevention messages.

The death toll associated with opioid overdose dramatically increased from 2017 to 2018 to over 1400 per year but due to the sustained efforts on reducing harm associated with the opioid crisis, they declined in 2019. However, the gains made in the last year maybe in jeopardy as the COVID-19 public health measures such as physical distancing may in effect encourage using alone and risk dying of overdose. In fact, the BC Coroner's monthly updates for March and April, 2020 point to a sharp increase in overdose deaths of 112 and 117 persons respectively compared to January and February where the numbers were below 80 (BC Coroners Services, 2020).

Furthermore, the spike in death is also possibly related to another COVID-related disruption; that of street supply chain from producers to end-users. As per the United Nations Office of Drugs and Crime (UNODC), the supply chain, from production, trafficking to end-use is likely to be affected due to the global shutdown of international borders and heighted security across borders (UNODC, 2020). The movement of street drugs heavily relies on the international trade activities and movements as it camouflages its operations under regulated and legal business entities (UNODC, 2020), hence a sharp decline of legal trade will impact the quantity and quality of street drugs. Furthermore, the dwindling supply of street drugs has already been felt and reported in the Vancouver DTES (Kelly, 2020). This shortage will have a domino effect on availability, quality, costs, risks of drug withdrawal, overdose as well as uptick in survival behaviors (criminal activities, sex work etc.).

With the opioid overdose mortality rate going up, there is fear of a spike in overdose again due to the effects of the corona virus. Hence, a double whammy for persons who use drugs.

A glimmer of hope in the midst of a pandemic

Over the years, the DTES has been a battle ground, so to speak, in the fight for progressive drugs and addiction policies. A struggle that led to the opening of the first North American supervised drug consumption site. A fight that went all way the up to the Canadian Supreme Court (Small, 2012). That struggle for progressive policies was led by persons with lived experiences, community activists, and policy and research experts who strongly advocated for harm reduction policies, programs and interventions to reduce the health, social and economic impact of drug use. In the last few years especially in the context of contaminated supply chain, the campaign shifted to a call to the federal and provincial government to decriminalize individual drug use and safe supply in order to combat overdose, reduce stigma and criminalization of those using drugs. Such a policy will led to better health outcome for drug users as evidence by the Portuguese example; a country that led the world in decriminalizing individual drug use and declaring drug use as a public health issue rather than a criminal justice one (Greenwald, 2009).

Despite calls, campaigns, policy and research briefs and even a call from the now famed BC's Public Health Officer, Dr. Bonnie Henry for the decriminalization of drug use there was little appetite on the part of the Provincial and Federal governments (CBC News, 2019). But COVID-19 has changed the discussions at least in BC, where at least in the short term, the BC government has formally approved a safe supply policy and plan to supplement for street drugs. In other words, individuals who use drugs can have access to pharmaceutical grade heroine and stimulants substitute in British Columbia in order to dually address COVID-19 and drug overdose (BCCSU, 2020).

The change of heart at the provincial level appears to have been neccissated by the COVID-19 crisis, and the question now is whether such a bold move will lead to a permanent policy change in the fight for progressive harm reduction in BC. Time will tell.

References

BC Coroners Services. (2020). *Illicit drug toxicity in BC.* https://www2.gov.bc.ca/assets/gov/birth-adoption-death-marriage-and-divorce/deaths/coroners-service/statistical/illicit-drug.pdf

BC Government. (2016). *How the province is responding.* Retrieved May 30, 2020, from https://www2.gov.bc.ca/gov/content/overdose/how-the-province-is-responding

British Columbia Center on Substance Use. (2020). *Risk mitigation in the context of dual public health emergencies: interim clinical guidance.* British Columbia Center on Substance Use.

CBC News. (2019). *BC's top doctor calls for regulated opioid supply after almost 1,500 deaths in 2018.* https://www.cbc.ca/news/canada/british-columbia/bonnie-henry-opioid-deaths-1.5009950

Greenwald, G. (2009). Drug decriminalization in Portugal: Lessons for creating fair and successful drug policies. Cato Institute Whitepaper Series. https://www.cato.org/publications/white-paper/drug-decriminalization-portugal-lessons-creating-fair-successful-drug-policies

Kelly, A. (2020). Dwindling drug supply in DTES drives price up, leaves users desperate as COVID-19 closes border. *CityNews 1130.* https://www.citynews1130.com/2020/03/24/drug-supply-bc-covid-19-border/

NIDA. (2019). *Fentanyl.* Retrieved May 30, 2020, from https://www.drugabuse.gov/publications/drugfacts/fentanyl on.

Small, D. (2012). Canada's highest court unchains injection drug users; implications for harm reduction as standard of healthcare. *Harm Reduction Journal, 9*(1), 34. https://doi.org/10.1186/1477-7517-9-34

UNODC. (2020). *COVID-19 and the drug supply chain: from production and trafficking to use.* United Nations Office of Drugs and Crime.

Finding Our Power Together: Working with Indigenous Youth and Children during COVID-19

Nicole Ineese-Nash

Indigenous communities continue to be under-resourced, under-funded, and overly managed and policed (Greenwood et al., 2012), which has only been exacerbated by COVID-19. Our ability to choose our own path has been gated, leaving only a singular paved road toward the center; toward assimilation. For many, this is not a choice at all. When young people are faced with the impossibility of thriving in poverty, through intergenerational and first-hand trauma, and without adequate resources to overcome these difficulties, they may choose to assert their agency in the only way they know how – by ending the journey altogether. Indigenous communities in northern parts of Canada have been experiencing an increase in youth suicide since 2011, according to a Statistics Canada report on First Nations, Inuit and Metis youth suicide (2019). Suicide and self-inflicted injuries are the leading cause of death for First Nation youth and adults (Public Health Agency of Canada, 2016). Young people (those under 25 years of age) also represent a significant percentage of the population in Indigenous communities, ranging from 40 to 80% (Statistics Canada, 2019). In addition, within this population, youth living on-reserve have higher rates of suicide than young people living off-reserve, due to the deeper feelings of social isolation, health disparities, and lack of connection to the outside world (Statistics Canada, 2019). This population has one of the highest growth rates in the world.

If young people continue to be born into a legacy of colonialism, into the systemic oppression of Indigenous sovereignty, and without appropriate or effective access to mental health support, medical care, or educational opportunities, we will surely see a steady increase in the number of deaths in our communities. These conditions have existed long before the COVID-19 pandemic, and will likely persist as we transition back to a more 'normal' way of living. However, 'normal' has never been adequate for Indigenous people in Canada; there is nothing 'normal' about young people taking their own lives in order to escape their colonial reality.

COVID-19 will undeniably impact Indigenous communities. In the short term, many communities are forced to make difficult decisions about how to keep their members safe, often at a great financial cost. Lockdowns are being employed as a safeguarding measure in many communities, which limits the transmission of infectious disease from external sources but also means that many community members are relying on provisional support from tribal governments. The processes of accessing federal funding structures to support communities in responding to COVID-19 have been difficult to navigate for many communities who do not have access to high-speed internet and there have been few mechanisms in place to support community leaders in completing the designated forms provided by Indigenous Services Canada. This has led to a delay in accessing vital provisions, such as Personal Protective Equipment (PPE) and testing kits. In the context of an unprecedented health crisis, time can be the deciding factor of community-wide transmission or mitigation.

While communities across Canada continue physical distancing measures, schools and community programs have shuttered and adapted to online delivery models. For Indigenous communities, however, this is difficult if not impossible to provide without increased infrastructure in place. In Nibinamik First Nation, for instance, a community of around 400 residents (80% of which are under the age of 40), very few young people have access to electronic devices in order to avail themselves of online education systems or mental health supports. Those that do have a device would still have difficulty accessing online programs due to limited and unstable internet connections. The Ontario government has sought to support access to electronic devices to students within the provincial education system (Ontario Ministry of Education, 2020), however, due to jurisdictional oversight of Indigenous education as a federal responsibility, there has been little discussion of how this type of support would be provided to First Nation communities. Online programming is often employed as a placeholder for investment in Indigenous education programs on reserve, particularly for remote or fly-in communities. However, these models can be difficult for Indigenous students to navigate and often rely on didactic modes of knowledge transmission that conflict with Indigenous pedagogies and worldviews that are more relational and experientially based. We know this means that many children and youth will not have access to any formal educational content while in isolation. Social isolation, which has been a long-term issue in many First Nations and a leading cause of youth suicide, is now exacerbated by mitigation measures.

Many young people are living in multi-generational homes that may be overcrowded, without access to clean water, telephone, or internet. Some young people may also be living in precarious arrangements with family members, foster caregivers, and acquaintances or may be caregiving for an elder or child themselves. Schools and community programs can provide a lifeline for Indigenous youth who may be experiencing mental health challenges; they serve as a mechanism to enter into the mental health service system. Without these critical relationships, many youth will have difficulty getting through this pandemic and will face long-term challenges in order to regain a strong sense of grounding in their lives. Unfortunately, some may not overcome these challenges.

Anishinaabe worldviews, cultures, and lifeways are premised on overcoming hardship. From struggle, we learn new ways of being, of surviving, and of thriving. I anticipate that this time will open us up for radical possibilities of relating to one another on a global scale; we can create a new 'normal' together. Many communities are returning to more traditional communal ways of being through reciprocal caregiving and a prioritization of social welfare over economic expansion. Young people are returning to the land as a way to sustain themselves and their communities. There is potential for developing new programs that prioritize Indigenous perspectives and circumstances, which may be beneficial to other communities. Funding structures may adapt to fill the gaps that have persisted long before this crisis emerged. Young people are taking up their roles as oshkabewisuk, or helpers, in their communities, guiding the way forward and forging new potentialities outside of the singular colonial existence. No one can be sure of what the future holds after COVID-19, but we do know that we will emerge from this stronger if we act in solidarity. Support for Indigenous youth in this unprecedented time allows for us to see and walk a good path together. It allows us to find our power together.

References

Greenwood, M. L., Leeuw, D., & Naomi, S. (2012). Social determinants of health and the future wellbeing of Aboriginal children in Canada. *Paediatrics and Child Health*, *17*(7), 381–384.

Ontario Ministry of Education. (2020). *News release. Ontario establishes key partnerships to make home learning more accessible iPad devices with free Rogers wireless data will support learning at home.* https://news.ontario.ca/edu/en/2020/04/ontario-establishes-key-partnerships-to-make-home-learning-more-accessible.html

Public Health Agency of Canada. (2016). *Suicide prevention framework.* https://www.canada.ca/en/public-health/services/publications/healthy-living/suicide-prevention-framework.html

Statistics Canada. (2019). https://www150.statcan.gc.ca/n1/pub/99-011-x/99-011-x2019001-eng.htm

Advocating for Health and Well-Being

Sara Jassemi

Between bites over lunch during an on-call week, I log on to our biweekly departmental meeting (over everyone's new favorite, Zoom, of course). Slides demonstrating improving epidemiological data and sober plans to reopen our communities and our hospital flash past. I feel a sense of hope that we are recovering on the whole, and then I am interrupted. I pick up the phone and consult with a colleague about a shared patient with a long-standing history of an eating disorder and trauma-related symptoms. There are some new and some familiar physical symptoms, and the patient and their parents are asking for direction. We've tried to space out in-person medical visits due to the COVID-19 pandemic, but this patient and family have needed consistent containment and support. Now, this patient may need an admission if they are medically unstable. As I work out the mental math of when we can arrange a new admission, I look down at my list of current inpatients, a crew of adolescents with complications from eating disorders and severe substance use disorders. Over the last few weeks, my subspecialty's list has grown just as long, or sometimes longer, than the general pediatrics Clinical Teaching Units' lists, which is unprecedented for our hospital. I observe a pattern. In front of me and on the phone were the diverse secondary effects of the COVID-19 pandemic on the mental and physical health of adolescents and their families. I am an Adolescent Medicine Pediatrician in Vancouver, Canada, specializing in the growth, development, and mental health of teenagers, and since the COVID-19 pandemic hit, we have been busier than ever.

In a recent Stanford University Pediatrics Grand Rounds, Dr. Lisa Chamberlain discussed the direct and indirect effects of the COVID-19 pandemic. Indirect effects of this unprecedented dual public health and economic crisis are biproducts of shelter in place, including increasing rates of unemployment and disruption in education. In British Columbia, where I work, we are living through a third concurrent crisis: the ongoing opioid crisis, which was declared a public health emergency in 2016. While the pediatric population has been fortunately spared from some of the harshest direct effects of COVID-19, the indirect effects are present, from the closure of community centers and programming to food insecurity. Moreover, health care providers are noticing that the pandemic is amplifying the stratification in the social determinants of health, and, as a result, there is a widening gap in health outcomes.

There might be more to this story. Yes, I see a divergence in health outcomes and the indirect effects of the pandemic between different patients of mine, and yes, most of the time, those groups are separated by disparities in the social determinants of health. But, there is another variable. I have seen the COVID-19 pandemic reveal the impact of 'family health' as a determinant of individual child and adolescent health. I use the term 'family' broadly to include parents, guardians, and trusted adults in the adolescent's extended family and community. I use the term 'health' to mean functioning within the family system as well as the mental and physical health of family members. Expressions of strong family health that I've seen include secure attachment, functional interpersonal communication, and caregivers' adaptive coping skills. Evidence of challenged family health includes adverse childhood events, violence, and caregiver maladaptive coping skills such as substance misuse.

This contrast was illustrated when two young adolescents with similar psychosocial and historical backgrounds presented to our emergency department recently with non-fatal fentanyl overdoses. Our hospital offers a stabilization admission to adolescents presenting with life threatening overdoses to provide motivational interviewing, initiation of opioid agonist therapy (OAT) if appropriate, opportunistic medical and psychiatric care, and a cohesive discharge plan. Since the pandemic began, emergency presentations for severe substance use disorders and overdoses in our hospital alone have doubled. Of the two adolescents, one elected to stay in hospital for a stabilization care admission and, unfortunately, one left against medical advice after a brief stay in the emergency department. The youth who was discharged from the emergency department left only with their group home workers and a phone call placed to the after-hours ministry worker. We arranged an outpatient appointment with an addiction medicine clinic, but I worry about the likelihood of follow-up given that most clinics only offer virtual health care visits at this time. It was already a challenge to engage this young person when we were in the same room together. I also worry about the health implications for this young person. The BC Coroners Service reported that approximately 30% of youth with fatal overdoses had a previous nonfatal overdose, a pattern seen similarly in adults.

In contrast, the youth who stayed was successfully re-initiated on their OAT, a life-saving intervention, and was discharged with ongoing age-appropriate, substance use follow-up. At the time of admission, this young person was with their group home workers, but they knew their grandparent would be there the next day and would remain by their side in hospital. There was a continuum of engaged family support, such as that grandparent who modeled healthy strategies by taking breaks when their own self-care was needed. Their child protection worker was far from burnt out, demonstrating compassion and attention and going above and beyond their usual duties. They were creative, flexible and attentive. In turn, this youth responded positively and collaboratively with the hospital staff and their supports. Reflecting on this admission, the health of this young person's *family* directly contributed to their health outcomes and their access to state-of-the-art medical care.

In my eating disorders clinic, I look forward to the regular virtual health phone visits I have with the parent of a young adolescent with avoidant-restrictive food intake disorder and social anxiety. Before the COVID-19 pandemic, this was a patient encounter that I would dread because I struggled to find the balance of emphasizing the urgency of weight restoration while also being mindful of the impact on their anxiety. Since shelter in place, a major stressor has been eliminated for this young patient: the social pressures of school. However, not only was a stressor taken away, something positive was also added. Shelter in place deepened the positive relationship between parent and child, which has resulted in weight restoration, vertical growth, and pubertal development in my patient and, from what I infer from our phone conversations, engagement and happiness in the parent. This is a lower-resourced family that might have been expected to have poor health outcomes due to their current social determinants of health. Yet, here what emerges is the health of the family relationships and the positive impact this has had on anxiety and eating behaviors.

Health is deeply influenced by our historical, societal, political, and economic environments. One level down in Bronfenbrenner's ecological model are the concentric circles of trusted family and community members embracing the adolescent patient who is at the center. When the family is healthy, and with appropriate supports, then the adolescent thrives. By removing outside influences and asking families to shelter at home, the COVID-19 pandemic shines a light onto the health not only of our individual patients, but on the health and functioning of their family systems. As health care providers to children and adolescents, we should be humbled and empowered with this knowledge. It is our imperative to see to and advocate for the health and well-being of our individual patients *and* that of their families.

Covid-19 and Intergenerational Anxiety and Trauma

Cecilia M. Jevitt

In the 1980s, I worked for the US Federal Community and Migrant Health Service in Florida. Our Birthing Team included midwives, obstetricians, a case management nurse, a social worker and Spanish-speaking community resource workers. The program was designed to improve perinatal outcomes through health and parenting education, shared decision making to reduce maternal and family stress and support arranged by the social worker. The prime directive of the community resource workers was, "*No asustes a la mama*," they cautioned over and over, "*o trendra un bebe nerviosa.*" "Don't scare the mother or you'll get a nervous baby." Any bad news or shock could cause *el susto*, the fright. *El susto* was sometimes dismissed as just the traditional way for rural Mexicans to manage anxiety.

Almost 40 years later, multiple research studies affirm that if you scare the mother, you get a nervous baby. The COVID-19 pandemic is hard to top as a source of *el susto*. At the start of the epidemic, the effect of the coronavirus during pregnancy to mother and fetus was unknown. Many viral respiratory illnesses such as measles, are known to affect pregnant women more seriously than those who are not pregnant, and many including the Zika virus can cause permanent damage to the fetus. For most, COVID-19 was a moderate to severe respiratory illness. Deaths in reproductive age women are small with 0.8% of adults ages 25–34 and 1.8% for those ages 35–44 dying after coronavirus infection. The death rate jumps to 12% at age 55, 21% at 65 and 30% at age 85 heightening fears in younger women. Case analyses from China demonstrated no increase in illness severity during pregnancy with little evidence that COVID-19 crosses the placenta; however, there are documented cases of in utero infection, immediate postpartum transmission of coronavirus from an infected mother to the newborn and COVID-19 has been isolated from breast milk. Learning to fear for the child is a developmental task of pregnancy but recent qualitative research in British Columbia shows that COVID-19 generates fears and uncertainty that cannot be calmed because of the incomplete knowledge about coronavirus in pregnancy.

Current research investigates three causative lines for childhood anxiety: genetic inheritance, intrauterine epigenetic changes to the hypothalamic–pituitary–adrenocortical axis (HPA axis), and postpartum disruptions to effective parenting in the maternal–newborn dyad. There is evidence of specific genes associated with anxiety and depression but new epigenetic research broadens potential mood priming mechanisms. The main output of the HPA axis, cortisol, is elevated during stress and anxiety. Women who are shocked, anxious, or chronically depressed have hypothalamic-pituitary-adrenal axis changes including chronically elevated cortisol levels that may hormonally prime the fetus for anxiety and depression by methylating genes and changing gene function to alter fetal HPA reactivity. Anxiety and depression might be more primed than inherited, starting even before the newborn meets the home-parenting environment.

Maternal anxiety and depression can affect more than the next generation. A female fetus forms all the eggs she will have for life while in her mother's uterus. Those eggs are subject to the same epigenetic changes that the fetus experiences. A scared grandmother can prime a female grandchild for anxiety. In addition to fear for self, newborn, family and friends from the disease, the COVID-19 pandemic-associated recession imposes unemployment with ensuing loss of income, food insecurity and for many, loss of housing. In the US, these COVID-19 associated stresses imposed on the day-to-day stresses of racism, and education, housing, and employment inequities may account for increased disease and death rates among blacks and Hispanics exposed to coronavirus. Although the data are incomplete, in many states the case and death rates for black and Hispanics are 2–4 times higher than those of whites are.

Before the COVID-19 pandemic, the incidence of maternal postpartum depressive and anxiety disorders were approximately 10% and 20%, respectively. Preliminary COVID-19 related postpartum research shows that anxiety and depression have increased sharply, eroding maternal caregiving energy. Both maternal prenatal anxiety and emotional stress are associated with higher reaction intensity in children, higher negative emotionality, significantly higher rates of behavioral problems and lower prosocial behavior in children. A growing body of studies finds significant links between prenatal stress and anxiety and child development up to adolescence. The social isolation of the COVID-19 pandemic separates pregnant women from their social support systems and mental health resources. The isolation also denies women the enjoyment of celebratory pregnancy rituals: gender-reveal parties, baby showers, postpartum visits by family and friends to congratulate the parents and meet the newborn. Early in the isolation, maternity care providers worldwide moved to the World Health Organization's limited prenatal care visit schedule. Any visits that could be provided by phone or video-conferencing were accomplished at a distance, limiting the support that could be provided during prenatal care. Hospitals moving to limit coronavirus transmission prevented women from having partners, family members or doulas with them in labor. Known supportive others have been demonstrated to shorten phases of labor and increase rates of uncomplicated vaginal birth.

What are the summative effects of the grand COVID-19 *susto*? Increased maternal and family anxiety and depression during the perinatal period and infants of two generations at risk for compromised parenting, anxiety and childhood depression. Social Work has an indispensable role in ameliorating the effects of the COVID-19 *susto*, by providing increased prenatal support for the mother and the family, securing support for food and housing, promoting family companionship for women during labor and birth, assuring easy access to counseling and mental health services, and early assessment of parenting and infant development. Analysis of data from Denmark, a country known for its accessible health care and social services, reports a 70% reduction in preterm labor and low birth weight newborns following two months of COVID-19 lockdown. Researchers have various explanations for these reductions but most include increased maternal rest, time with families that reduces stress, and a broad social safety net. Denmark may be a living lab in the analysis of the effects of accessible health care and social services during a pandemic. While medicine searches for a COVID-19 cure, social work can bridge the immediate needs of the *susto* and the lasting risk for anxiety and depression two generations forward.

The Longer-Term Ramifications of the Covid-19 Pandemic for Children, Families, and Their Communities

Daniel Ji and Grant Charles

In this article, we present our thoughts on the longer-term ramifications of the Covid-19 pandemic for children, families, and their communities in Canada. Covid-19 has significantly disrupted future prospects for children and teens educationally, socially, and emotionally. For many children, school is about more than learning the curriculum; there are wraparound services provided through school such as speech-language and social work support, classroom behavioral and learning aides, multicultural support, and psychological services that are crucial to helping many children meet their developmental needs. Children who can no longer access these vital services due to school closures may experience negative consequences like teasing and bullying from other children as well as exclusion. These consequences may, in turn, lead to acting out or internalizing behavior. In short, losing months of school is disproportionately detrimental for educationally vulnerable children, and online schooling is an inadequate long-term solution. Furthermore, interactions at school are critical developmentally because children learn the skills necessary to form and maintain adult relationships. Children who are socially isolated for an extended period of time now may have an increased probability of becoming socially isolated later, and the redemptive measures to follow may be a case of too little, too late. For these reasons, among others, we may see a significant spike in diagnoses of mental illness among children and adolescents for prolonged stress after Covid-19, along with a host of coping mechanisms used to deal with its aftermath.

A vital factor contributing to many teenagers' prospects of postsecondary education is being able to save money through part-time or summer employment. Covid-19 is resulting in many business closures, significantly constraining employment possibilities and, by extension, curbing postsecondary prospects for many youths in the longer term. It is likely that even parents wishing to support their children financially so that they can attend college or trade school have been negatively financially impacted themselves. There are at least two possible implications: First, many young people will not be able to obtain employment that requires postsecondary education or may be significantly delayed in doing so with student loan debt posing a formidable challenge. Second, young people will have to become creative in how they secure an income and acquire marketable skills.

Provincial and federal governments have touted the strength of Canada's supply chains to discourage panic buying of food and supplies. However, the Covid-19 pandemic is a unique and protracted situation that may result in shifts that could become hard to pull back in the longer term. Supply line diversions overseas over an extended period of time could lead to greater insecurity of foods such as beef that may trickle down to compound the stress already experienced by families. The task of securing nutritious food and supplies may constitute a formidable challenge to families already under duress. The stress from Covid-19 is unlike stress caused by major disasters or armed conflicts. It is an ever-present, low-level slow burn. Children unaccustomed to dealing with such anxiety rely on their parents and caregivers to make sense of life during the pandemic and likely after as well. However, even when parents are doing a good job of helping their children manage anxiety, the anxiety is still present. It is a situation that parents may have a hard time explaining to their children, and a harder time still to make promises about when it will end.

In this new world with Covid-19, taxed parents may be either directly or unintentionally teaching fearfulness of others to their children. For example, one experience with which both writers are familiar has been pulling back responses from children walking with their parents in the local community. The seeds of paranoia being sown by well-intentioned parents may have longer-term ramifications for these children in adulthood. Stigmatization of individuals who have an easily visible illness is unfortunate enough on its own, but how do we prepare children for an environment where the virus is highly contagious, yet symptoms possibly mild or even nonexistent? If Covid-19 carriers can be asymptomatic, and even some symptoms may be confused for spring allergies or other minor illnesses, wariness or paranoia of others rooted in persistent, low-level anxiety could have lasting effects on children, youth, and families. Potential adverse reactions to crowded places, fear of contamination, overly frequent hand washing, generalized fear of leaving the house, and potential health anxiety and misinterpretation of bodily cues as illness are all potential unprecedented longer-term ramifications. In the search to identify a scapegoat, xenophobia and racism toward Asians may become rampant.

The reasonable vigilance being practiced now by families may become maladaptive hypervigilance as the pandemic continues.

Returning to the beginning, the pandemic has shone a light on the inadequacies of our current systems designed to provide care and inclusion for children and their families. Life after Covid-19 may be a time for us as a society to prioritize and then deliver the services and programs that consider paramount the developmental needs of all children in family and community environments to help them thrive. We may have a chance to see the need left by Covid-19 for free postsecondary education for the sake of a brighter future. Perhaps we may even have an opportunity to reflect on who gets to define what type of work is essential given our great needs in this challenging hour, and provide living wages with benefits to those who have met our needs in spite of the risks to themselves and their own families. Rather than pulling away from each other in fear or hate, perhaps we can pull together as a society to learn from our failings and commit to bettering the lives of our children, teens, families, and communities.

The Crisis of Loss and Moral Injury – Lasting Effects of COVID-19 on Teenagers and Healthcare Workers

Richard La Fleur

For many people around the world, Coronavirus (COVID-19) may have lasting effects that reshape human behavior and interaction both locally and collectively. While there are immediate changes to how we relate to each other from a societal perspective (social distancing) and the role of leaders and government in our lives, there are also changes that will have long lasting effects on our future (preparedness for the next global event) that will not be fully understood for some time.

As a psychologist, I have noticed a shift in human behavior, including an increase in individual and institutional levels of fear and anxiety along with misperceptions of reality and reasoning. In this article, I will be addressing fear and anxiety through the lens of teenagers who are directly affected by COCID-19–(dealing with loss) and how healthcare workers respond to the events of COVID-19, more specifically how they are affected by Moral Injury–possibility of lingering effects on family life.

Teenagers and Coping with Loss

A few weeks ago, I was honored to be part of an Instagram Live session with approximately 40 teenagers who had questions about the current pandemic. During our time together a graduating senior asked a question, then made a statement that was not only important but also relevant to the times. Her question was, "*why did this have to happen now*"? While this may seem to be a self-serving question (and maybe it was), her follow-up statement put everything into perspective for me. Her statement was–"*I have not stopped to process everything that is happening around me, and right now in this moment, I feel as though I lost a part of my life.*" It was at this moment I realized our teenagers have not been able to process the losses they are currently experiencing, nor are they equipped to cope with loss.

To better understand the effects of loss, we must first understand what it means to be attached. Turning to the work of John Bowlby, attachment helps provide safety and security in human development. The classroom and the structure of school (for many students) is a place of familiarity as well as a place of safety (for the most part) and security. At school, many milestones are celebrated in the classroom (birthdays, lost tooth, new pets, driver's license), learning and loving are moments that are shared with the anticipation of nine months of growing together.

Students become attached to the school calendar because it is set in stone and only the coveted snow day could alter its existence. They are also attached to the rhythm of their day as they change classes and linger in the hallways, operating in chaotic symphony–but it is their day! And what about the graduating senior, who worked hard and diligently to get to this 'rite of passage' of preparing for the senior trip, or walking across the stage to be handed the well-deserved High School Diploma or getting dressed up in a tuxedo or a gorgeous evening dress, ready to attend prom with the person they dreamt of for years! What happens when these precious and anticipated moments are taken away in a single day? "Ok, I'll see you guys on Monday, have a good weekend"! But Monday never came …

How does a teenage mind, one that still does not have the ability to fully engage the frontal cortex, process these deep and meaningful losses? As adults, we have different skills and life experiences that hopefully gives us what we need to process life, even when it does not make sense–but what about our teenagers? Losses of this magnitude have both long-term and short-term effects on the family unit as well as the community they are a part of. While I was on the Instagram Live session with students, they were expressing feelings of sadness, anger, anxiety and loneliness. They were genuinely struggling with where they are in life and while loss is universal and the sting of loss can be devastating for many, for some teenagers, COVID-19 seems like an endless nightmare that they cannot wake up from.

Healthcare Workers and Moral Injury

On another front, one area of deep concern for me is the after effects of COVID-19 on our healthcare workers. I recently heard an interview given by a psychiatrist who stated that many healthcare workers will suffer from PTSD, similar to Vietnam veterans and military personnel, postwar or deployment. While I believe there will be increases in the number of PTSD cases, I also believe there will be a higher increase in the unseen wounds–the wounds of Moral Injury.

Recently, Moral Injury has gained some traction in literature and research, but it has not been fully conceptualized nor understood. For some researchers and practitioners, Moral Injury is closely connected to PTSD and while there may be some overlap between the two, Moral Injury holds its own structure and is directly connected to a person's belief system. In its simplest form, Moral Injury is the inability to reconcile one's own belief with a morally injurious act. To go a bit further, Moral Injury is–*giving consent to or agreeing to or failing to prevent an immoral act, witnessing or learning about acts that transgress deeply held moral beliefs and personal standards* (Litz et al., 2018).

With this definition in mind, many of our healthcare workers (technicians, nurses, doctors and staff) are currently caring for those who are suffering from COVID-19 and due to the current state of healthcare systems (overloaded and reduced resources), many healthcare workers are making decisions that directly affect human life. For some it is a matter of choice–who lives and who dies due to the severity of this pandemic. Death and the process of dying (in some cases inhumane) seems to be a normal outcome from COVID-19. I think it is safe to say, death is a natural part of this life but excessive and abnormal death is not something anyone could be prepared for.

With this in mind, healthcare workers were faced with the added responsibility of attending to family members who were unable to be with their loved ones. In this same vein, they became extensions of the family–the human interface to relay final thoughts, wishes, prayers and messages of love to those who were in their last moments of life. Moral Injury is inevitable. It is safe to say our healthcare workers are living and working in morally injurious times. With this thought in mind, many of our healthcare workers will be considered *Suffering Souls*–unable to reconcile their morality. The inability to be reconciled to one's morality happens as time passes by. As humans, we engage in the process of hindsight, we look back in time and ask questions such as, "How could I?, we ask, What was I thinking? If only .... These are the sorts of moments we want back, only to arrive at the harsh and terrible realization that they are gone forever (Freeman, 2010). This can be especially troubling in the sphere of moral life. Our position is different and our morals seem different than when we acted or when we did not.

For me, these are two crucial topics and populations who need us and the various interventions to help create healing environments. These are important concepts to discuss because there will be many suffering souls after COVID-19. Our teenagers and our healthcare workers deserve as much as we can give. I have found by engaging in an intervention called Just-Listening, which provides a non-judgmental environment for people to share and express their thoughts. Just-Listening is a safe space where healing can occur.

References

Freeman, M. (2010). *Hindsight: The promise and peril of looking backward.* Oxford University Press.

Litz, B., et al. (2018). *Adaptive disclosure: A new treatment for military trauma, loss, and moral injury.* The Guildford Press.

COVID-19: Effects of the Shutdown on Children and Families in Child and Youth Care Services in Germany

Maya Lorch and Dunja Fuchs

Aside from the general effects of the restrictions that everybody experiences to a different degree, including the need to find ways to bring structures into daily life and to balance the parents' job demands with care and homeschooling, children living in child and youth care services find themselves in special circumstances. This is evident in both the short and long term ramifications of the pandemic for children and youth living in our residential programs under the auspices of municipal child and youth services.

The children of residential groups are not allowed to have any face-to-face contact with their parents. This is especially difficult for children who have just been transferred into long-term residential services and for those who have a strong emotional bond to their parents. This aspect is also challenging for the staff on various levels: the administration has to balance safety issues against the legal rights of parents and their children to see each other regularly. And the staff in residential programs have to explain these decisions and to respond to the frustrations, anger and grief that they bring for the children.

In these emotionally challenging situations, structures and routines are crucial for children, as they provide orientation and stability – particularly for children with deficits in their emotional regulation. With the loss of the normal daily life structures and routines, many of our children have lost their outer (or external) navigational system, which usually is a means for inner orientation and self-regulation. This is evidenced by an overall sensitivity and a tendency to be irritated more easily. In the future, this could solidify as a general anxiousness in some children, making them either emotionally dependent on external structures or refusing the scaffold of outer norms altogether. Both scenarios may impede the development toward a healthy and functioning member of society. The fact that there is no transparent exit (or discharge) strategy and that the programs can only plan and act on a week-to-week basis increases the feelings of insecurity for all parties involved, including management, staff, children and parents.

Another ramification especially for the children in our care is that they are only allowed to leave the group homes under adult supervision. As a consequence, they are constantly together with the other young people of their group but they have no chance of meeting their individual friends. This could have a long-term impact on their friendships and networks outside of child and youth services. It also runs counter to what residential services have been proactively addressing for some time now by promoting decentralized structures and signing up young people living in residential care for mainstream recreational activities and sports clubs. Furthermore, the constant adult supervision, together with the avoidance of public transportation, is undermining efforts of increasing the independence of the children. In some cases, this may lead to a general cautiousness or even a regressing of a previously achieved autonomy.

Homeschooling creates a particular challenge for residential groups. Groups with eight children of different ages are usually staffed with one caregiver, who obviously cannot help all children simultaneously. This is especially difficult as all the children work on different tasks and many of the children have learning difficulties and/or problems with motivation and concentration. Furthermore a technical problem makes home schooling more difficult: there is no Wi-Fi in the residential groups and limited computers. Even the quickly distributed tablets (one for each group) can only be used under supervision. Therefore, all worksheets have to be printed even if they could be completed online and finished tasks can only be sent to the teachers on paper. This leads to a rather delayed feedback from the teachers whereas these young people need a direct and quick response to their efforts. All of this tends to harden the stereotype that children from residential groups are slow learners and are not looked after and supported enough. A long-term consequence could be that the gap between our and 'problem free' young people gets bigger, leading to an even higher need of supportive systems.

In spite of the many negative effects listed above, . we experience a lot of solidarity in different forms and at various levels:

- People from inside and outside our services sewed and donated hundreds of masks for children and staff alike;
- The management provided tablets and portable Wifi-cubes for home schooling to all groups, as well as vouchers for a weekly pizza-delivery;
- Coworkers from other departments of child and youth care services are helping to compensate for the increased demands of care;

- In the groups, we see a higher identification with the group itself together with a stronger positive dynamic among the children;
- The staff have more time and open space to interact more intimately with the children and youth: things like cooking, playing games and reading together can be done more often and in a more relaxed manner.

In summary, all the challenges associated with the pandemic lead to higher levels of stress for everybody and we can see that conflicts, both amongst young people and between young people and adults, escalate more quickly. In the short-term, all parties involved try to manage within their capabilities. The long-term effects remain to be seen. While we hope that some of the positive developments and experiences during this pandemic will contribute to resilience and long-term growth for the young people, and perhaps even to the well being of our organization, the reality is that some things may have lasting impacts that are less positive. We don't really know what the consequences of family separation will be; we don't know how the limited opportunities to exercise autonomy will impact young people beyond the short-term; and we also don't know the extent to which some of the challenges associated with the young people's schooling may create gaps and greater challenges in the months and years ahead. For right now, everybody endeavors to make the best of the situation and to stick it out together.

Engagement Redefined: Children and Youth without parental Care during and post Covid-19, India

Kiran Modi and Leena Prasad

Children already in vulnerable situations and difficult circumstances in normal times are always at the threshold of a crisis. Even before coming to alternative settings, children in out of home care have already experienced early childhood trauma, deprivations of all kinds, met with human depravity of different shades. The slightest trigger can send them to critical re-traumatization. To be able to prevent this, in the face of the rising issues caused by this pandemic, right assessments, effective interventions and working to keep the trust of children with their care givers is of paramount importance.

Udayan Care, an NGO in India, headquartered in Delhi, manages 17 group homes for children (Udayan Ghars: Sunshine Homes) and two after-care facilities for youth. We also support a care leavers association for vulnerable children and youth.

It is a huge task for all the social workers, counselors and administrative staff at Udayan Care to reach out to the over 200 children and 30 youth, who are directly under our care and protection, and the over 50 care leavers in two different cities. We need to ensure that they do not lose their voice, do not feel forgotten, do not experience any heightened negative feelings or anxious moments and that they also feel gainfully engaged as lock-down does not permit us, other than the skeletal residential staff, to be physically present at the facilities,

The first steps we implemented involved stopping outsiders from visiting the homes, training children and staff in remaining home bound and to observe safe distancing. This meant that almost all the volunteers and professionals had to stay away from their beloved children and youth. Our residential care staff picked up the cudgels and have stood bravely to face the call of duty. It has been heartening to not only see them keeping children well-fed, well sanitized, and engaged positively in a routine developed together with the children and youth but also quickly adapting to technology to keep connected with the mentors, and other professional staff.

The key has been to keep children engaged. The crisis brought by Covid-19 has given the mentor parents, social workers and the caregivers at homes a chance to be closer to their children and youth even more than they could during normal times. Close conversations even online have definitely increased the trust in each other, showing that life and what we have in life must not be taken for granted. This has helped children see the positive side even in this tough situation as is evident in the words of a 14 year old girl, Sheelu: "this Corona has taught me how to look after my other sisters in the home so that they don't feel anxious, for my questions on anxiety are so nicely allayed by my counsellor; I feel confident that we will fight it together." Another youth remarked "With so much crisis in our country at this time due to the Corona virus, I may sound stupid to come out as happy, engaging myself a lot more than before with new online learning tools, as my Counselor *didi* (big sister) has told me to always stay positive and look for opportunities everywhere."

Finding the most appropriate and suitable care during this pandemic has involved an increased focus on health and hygiene, teaching and managing children remotely, managing work remotely and being able to stay connected virtually. These changes come with challenges. Keeping children engaged online for a long time may become a difficult task for child and youth care practitioners. One major concern for the 23.6 million children without parental care in India who may or may not be in institutions, is non-availability of access to technical resources. At this moment huge efforts are being made by schools and teachers to deliver tutorials online or through television broadcasts. Some institutions may be providing the necessary technology and equipment, but concerns are rising for the impending negative effects of home confinement and these online schooling measures on children's physical and mental health.

Evidence suggests with less physical activity, longer screen time, irregular sleep patterns, and less favorable diets, there will be a spike in weight gain and a loss of cardiovascular fitness. More neglected will be the attention to psycho-social support to children. With online counseling, that also has not been available immediately and regularly, the stressors like boredom, inability to meet peers and teachers, lack of privacy, worry about their own families back home, and peer abuse, can leave enduring effects on children and adolescents. With no clarity on how long the situation will last, there is also a general uncertainty. For those with huge trauma issues and with special needs, more virtual programmes and strategies will need to be developed to reduce their stress and not let them fall into the vicious cycle of re-traumatization.

The immediate repercussions of this crisis are already being felt. Managing human and financial resources efficiently will be the biggest cause of concern. With increased focus on humanitarian and relief work, funding for children who stay in institutions, which already was a low priority, will likely be further reduced. Being able to maintain the standards of care with limited budgets available will be the biggest concern most institutions are going to face.

Care leavers, who always had difficulty getting jobs, will be hugely deprived as compared to youth in India who may still have some family support. Lack of jobs will increase homelessness and other issues. We, as a society should start strategizing to overcome these impending challenges.

Going forward, we hope to continue to receive the same and perhaps more committed support from duty bearers, various state agencies, child protection functionaries on the ground, schools, communities and last but not the least our donors. With the long lasting adverse effects of Covid-19 on the global economy, we are already seeing a dip in donor commitments. Government will need to step in and support voluntary efforts. The education sector will need to think of innovative ways of social distancing while still keeping children connected and moving forward. More tele-counseling services will be needed. More innovative practices in fund raising will need to be developed to keep the cogs of the wheel well-oiled and running.

Finally, making the paradigm shift for institutional care toward successful family and community based care, to which India started committing itself more forcefully only recently, may take a dip for the time being. Increased poverty and loss of livelihoods will mean reduced capacities of families to care for their children and steps to prevent separation of children from their families and to support families and communities to keep their children, need to be taken with support systems in place and a lot of monitoring mechanisms. Any unplanned effort to reduce the reliance on institutions in the post-Covid era could lead to a rush to send the children back, even to dysfunctional families. This will not be in the best interest of children and will take a toll on the already inadequate service system.

In such uncertain times, the only certainty is the need to keep evolving and developing, for the sake of our children and youth!

Covid: What's Next for Indigenous People?

Marie Nightbird

Being asked to share some thoughts about *What comes next? Life After Covid-19* for Indigenous peoples in Canada led me on an emotional path. Feel free to join me as I recall this journey.

When reflecting on the question "*What comes next?*" a deep overwhelm emerged as feelings of loss, sadness, anger, and confusion surfaced, so I paused, took a breath, and focused on the present. It is here that I see entwined with a multitude of continuing and upcoming hardships and heartaches and what I believe will be the ending of many aspects of normalcy, that I also see the many layers of resilience, strength, community, creativity, and love come through yet again.

Pausing in the present and slowing scrolling through the numerous ways the pandemic hits Indigenous peoples differently and destructively, ways that my mind has at times struggled to understand and at other times intentionally pushed aside, I could see how the ongoing impacts of colonization exacerbate the impact of Covid-19 in many undeniable ways. There is absolutely no doubt in my mind that Covid-19 has impacted everyone differently. For Indigenous communities, the destructive differences encompass a range of challenges from living in communities where there is no clean water to practice one of the best safeguards known, to wash our hands; to living in overcrowded living arrangements where one cannot practice yet another promoted safeguard, to socially isolate; to having to work or study at home when many rural and remote Indigenous communities have limited Internet capacity and many are without laptops and printers, in both rural or urban settings. General, so-called "normal" anxiety about not getting Covid-19 is intensified with a high rate of chronic illnesses increasing vulnerability, when purchasing hand sanitizer is not a possibility due to location and/or finances, and when, for some, the recollection of the loss of far too many due to tuberculosis and small pox is triggered. Deep concern over the loss of elders, with many being one of the few who can share their language, their history, and their stories. Add to this the need to reach out to and rely upon the government for assistance, a relationship known to provide the exact opposite.

I scrolled further and considered the overrepresentation of Indigenous peoples in jails where social distancing is difficult if not impossible, and to the awareness that the high percentage of Indigenous people who access community resources have had access to these services limited, if not stopped, access to things including the basics such as food. Jobs have been lost in sectors where many youth find employment, such as restaurants. And as it is common for many Indigenous people with employment to assist family members, the impact of the loss of employment faced by one can often spread far to others.

I started to wonder why it has taken this pandemic for others to see that the basics—water, food, employment, and so on — are so fragile or nonexistent. Why ... the legacy of colonization continues ... the anger resurfaces.

Then there was the need to pause again, to see that along with, or in spite of, this is the legacy of our strength, our power, and our unity. This is shown in many ways, such as drumming, singing, smudging, and circles available on line (many elders are more tech savvy than I am!), with First Nations looking to old ways of isolation for protection and some Nations having checkpoint dances at the protective barriers created to protect their communities. There is also Metis utilizing YouTube to have a Michif word of the day to learn and various cultural activities to enjoy, and Inuvik families receiving Internet supports for at-home learning. I think about how some youth are able to spend more time with relatives and more time outside, and how some youth are partaking in opportunities to connect with others, to share, and to help, to see the need to continue to stand, to speak, and to shine.

My thoughts rolled to my mom, a woman in her late 80s, who had two emergency pacemakers inserted during the early stages of the pandemic. I have not seen her as she is in a very high-risk category; I have been ready to go numerous times, drawing upon strength from places unknown to not go. Over the past weeks we have had frequent telephone contact, laughed to the point of crying, I think a combination of both joy and sadness coming through as we figured out how to safely navigate things, from ordering medical equipment, to food, to socks, to helping her sort out her last wishes. I wondered how we are making it through this unforeseen situation, and I see we are doing it with humor, in silence as we both hold our phones (likely more silence for her as she has a hard time hearing), by sharing stories. One story she loves to share is one she describes a good childhood memory, which is when she and her sisters and her mom would receive a box of apples from relatives. She tells me about the aroma, the taste, the pleasure of having food, the kindness of relatives she did not know very well … I can almost taste an apple as she talks.

I left my pause in the present and returned to thinking about the future, about "*What comes next*" for Indigenous peoples in light of Covid-19. My journey led me to clearly see that I truly don't know what the future holds; I have such an overwhelming sense of uncertainty, loss, and hardships. But what I very clearly do believe is that our strength will continue to come through and carry us, strength seen in many different ways, including in the simple act of sharing, be it apples or something grander, to someone, to anyone as we are all impacted by Covid-19, now and in the future.

We are all in this together. Thanks for walking this path with me. All my relations.

Thanks for joining me on this path. All my relations.

Challenges for Indigenous Children and Youth

Ashley Quinn

While the Coronavirus (COVID 19) presents unique challenges to everyone in our Vancouver, Canada communities, these challenges are exasperated for Indigenous children and youth currently in and aging out of foster care, many of whom have gone missing or whose lives have been lost in the downtown east side. In March 2020, the provincial government announced 'stay at home orders', with the intention of slowing down the spread of COVID 19.

Vancouver community social programs shut their doors, such as Urban Butterflies and Mentor Me, which Indigenous children and youth involved in child welfare regularly rely on for various forms of cultural support and visits with their biological families. The drivers who Indigenous foster children, their foster parents and biological families depend on to attend regularly scheduled family visits and cultural programming have been laid off, compromising the trusting relationships they have worked hard to build. Almost overnight, stores closed and boarded up, schools and community programming were canceled and Indigenous youth in and aged out of care were faced with further isolation from their families and support systems, as a sense of normalcy and consistency in their lives was interrupted and rapidly ceased.

For the past 18 years through the Urban Butterflies program in Vancouver, Indigenous girls 7–16 years of age in foster care, have met biweekly to engage with Indigenous Elders, leaders and each other in unique and fun opportunities to learn traditional teachings and about their spirituality, cultural art and dance, and gain skills to survive emotional pain associated with living in foster care away from their families. Through their participation, girls acquire a greater awareness of how to reduce and prevent risk factors and improve their health outcomes as they form meaningful long-term relationships, learn skills to be self-reliant and know where to go for help and support.

Adhering to COVID-19 restrictions, Urban Butterflies has been canceled and this has had adverse effects on Indigenous girls in foster care, their biological families, their Elders and their leaders, some of whom are Mentor Me program members. Mentor Me is an extension of Urban Butterflies and is a monthly program for Indigenous young women, 17–25 years of age, who have aged out of foster care. Mentor Me is a safe haven and provides a much-needed support system through community activities and cultural projects that enhance their lives together and build their leadership skills. Mentor Me members make significant contributions to the lives of younger Indigenous girls currently in the foster care system by regularly facilitating the Urban Butterflies program, through their deep-rooted relationships with the girls and knowing the importance of having older role models and supportive adults who care and listen to them. Consequently, these program members have not been able to connect with each other, which is essential for bonding and sustaining these important relationships.

Urban Butterflies and Mentor Me are the only Indigenous programs in Vancouver specifically dedicated to meeting the cultural needs of Indigenous girls involved in the child welfare system and this is the first time in their history they have been canceled. For the first month of the 'stay at home' order, program leaders primarily focused on providing emotional support and meeting immediate needs by delivering medicine, food and toiletries. Youth aged out of care are on limited budgets and without transportation to food banks and affordable grocery stores, have been in serious need for food, especially fresh fruit, vegetables and protein. While doing their best to address immediate needs, program leaders are concerned about the devastating impacts on Indigenous children in foster care when they are not able to visit with their biological families or connect with each other through community cultural programming. For many youth involved in child welfare, isolation is not new and for some, it brings back negative memories and associations of abuse, trauma and poverty.

The initial shock started to fade and as we began to adjust to the reality of our 'new normal', the sense of extreme isolation and emotional fatigue set in. The first month turned into the second and program leaders continued to deliver food and medicine, and began to include gift cards, hand sanitizer, masks, books, art supplies and other activities. Special baskets were delivered during Easter weekend. Although the long-term impacts of COIVD-19 are yet to be realized, the current negative impacts are continuing to have rippling effects on the physical, emotional, mental and spiritual health of Indigenous girls in and aged out of foster care. The need to restructure the Urban Butterflies and Mentor Me programs in a way that follows social distancing protocols is evident; however, the route to achieve this with limited funding is less clear.

OPEN ACCESS

Covid-19 Fares Gently with Children and Youngsters, But They Bear a Large Burden Due to the Lock down of the Society

Charlotte Reedtz

Daily news headings like "We may all die" along with in-depth descriptions of how painful it is to die of pneumonia caused by COVID-19, has been the reality since March in Norway. As of now, we know a great deal about COVID-19. We know that most people who get sick, and who died from it, have one or more underlying illnesses and are elderly people. We know that around 80% of our population get no, few or mild symptoms when affected by the virus. We know that children and youngsters are affected in milder ways, with very few symptoms, and are not at risk of becoming seriously sick or dying. The latter is not only true for the Norwegian population, but worldwide. However, we know very little about the effects of the interventions that have been put in place to prevent the virus from spreading, especially those related to lock down of societies. This is especially true for children and youngsters. In my view, the lock down of Norway is far more costly for our around 1 million young citizens, than COVID-19 itself. There are several reasons for this.

In my view, the mass media have gone far in provoking fear and anxiety among people. This may affect young children hard, as they are not cognitively mature enough to make the distinction between fake news and facts. Children depend on their caregivers to get good explanations about viruses, pandemics and risks, and if caregivers are fearful and anxious themselves, this may affect the way they inform and talk to children about these matters. In Norway, several parents feared contamination to the degree that their young children were not allowed to play with children outside the family at all during the Lock down. After the daycare centers were allowed to open on April 20, 25% of parents still kept their children at home. Unwarranted fear and anxiety in children present a risk for several negative health outcomes.

In Norway, day care centers and schools were shut down for 5–6 weeks, against the advice from the Norwegian Institute of Public Health. Only children of parents in essential societal positions had access to child care services. For a long period of time, most to children were at home with their parents, many of who have had to work from home during the lock down. Numerous studies shows that students who are struggling in their learning often have parents who are unable to offer necessary support and help. Academically strong students often have parents with resources and are able to support the education of their offspring. Based on this, an implication of closing Schools is that weaker students runs the risk of lagging further behind, while stronger students most likely will keep up with the curriculum. There have also been reports of drop-outs from school, because of the lack of structure and face-to-face support many students need. A recent Norwegian survey among parents showed that 25% felt their children learned less during the school lock down and several surveys support this. Furthermore, exams were canceled for thousands of students, resulting in fewer opportunities to qualify for later study programs.

There is no doubt that a lack of school activities may result in poorer learning and a less optimal education for students, especially for those who need special education or strong social support from teachers. Social isolation from school may also have resulted in a lack of social support that many students would normally get in their school environments. Many students do not have friends to spend time with outside school hours, and hence lonely students may have felt even lonelier.

In addition, many parents have been temporarily laid off their work or have lost their jobs, and are, therefore under great distress. Financial hardship and poverty are risk factors for children, as such life circumstances tend to affect both physical, social and emotional variables that determine parental life quality, and hence also children's life quality. A large group of children in Norway also live with parents with substance abuse problems and mental disorders. The lock down of the society had significant consequences for children living under such conditions as support and interventions were also shut down. At the same time, the bars in Oslo were open, while schools were closed. The Wine Monopoly stores (state-owned liquor stores) were open every day of the lock down, and some of these even established services to bring the alcoholic beverages home to people. This has put children who are not receiving adequate care from their parents or extended family at even greater risk.

This relates to my last point of concern which, is that home is not a safe place for all. Many youngsters live in families with domestic violence, sexual, physical and emotional abuse, and neglect. Many of these children need protection and their families need support and help from child welfare services. The main goal of these services is to ensure that children and adolescents who are living under conditions that represent a risk to their health and/or development, receive the help they need when they need it, so that children and adolescents grow in safe, secure and caring conditions. Failure to provide adequate care is the most common reason for intervention from Public services. However, most of the service activities to support children and their families were shut down during the lock down in Norway.

Group-based parent training, home visits and other interventions offering social support were paused. Norwegian child protection services had large problems in recruiting new visitation families and foster families during the spring semester, even larger troubles than before. The number of children who receive assistance from the child welfare system because of neglect and abuse has been increasing in Norway during the last two decades. However, during April 2020 there was a large reduction in referrals to Child Welfare Services in general. There was also a 35% reduction of acute placements outside families in Norway, as well as a reduction of 36% of new placements outside the family compared to 2019. Court custody cases about children who need protection were canceled and postponed, thus leaving minors in unbearable life circumstances for an even longer time.

In my view, a child perspective is necessary to understand the harmful effects of the COVID-19 pandemic for the young citizens of Norway. The spring when you turned 16 will never come back. The year you graduated from high school will always be 2020, but this year it was without a ceremony or party. A corona slogan in Norway says "It will end well". However, NeXT year is not so relevant for youth, as they tend to live their life here and now. Some of them have a lot of fear. Many have had poorer learning outcomes and a weakened education. Too many children have been enduring inadequate care and support in their homes. The question that needs to be asked when summing up the costs of the lock down for minors is: Was it worth it?

COVID-19, the Opioid Epidemic and the Housing Crisis

Lydia Rezene

During my years as a Community Health Specialist, I have worked directly with individuals who face multiple barriers, including those who use drugs, people who experience homelessness and people living with high risk of contracting Hepatitis C and HIV. During COVID-19, my colleagues and I have been reassigned to support with essential services for our most vulnerable populations. As a result, we have seen firsthand how COIVD-19 has impacted our clients and the community. In this brief article, I will highlight my observations of and experiences with people who use drugs during the COIVD-19 pandemic.

The COVID 19 pandemic has affected each and every one of us in some capacity. At the community level, many concerns have been raised pertaining to issues of food security, mental health, economic pressures, personal safety and physical isolation. For the people we support, these challenges are exacerbated when they intersect with unfavorable social determinants of health, such as inadequate housing, food insecurity, financial need, access barriers to support services and underlying health issues. For people who use drugs, additional factors such as access to a safe supply of substances, level of dependency, safety and stigma can further elevate the risks and negative consequences of a pandemic.

During the Pandemic, the supply of drugs has decreased and along with it, the access to drugs. Some possible reasons for this include the decreased border crossings, stricter regulations on domestic travel as well as the communal nature of distributing drugs and its risk to personal safety. Given a decrease in supply, prices have increased for a range of drugs, such as heroin, cocaine and crystal meth. Safe and affordable drug supplies are becoming harder to find and a number of clients have reported barriers to accessing their regular suppliers, forcing them to navigate unfamiliar avenues to obtain substances. Despite this, front line workers in one overdose prevention site in the Toronto's downtown core have reported higher usage rates among both dependent and recreational users and a significant hike in overdoses.

One strategy often used to expand supply is cutting product potencies by mixing in higher doses of sedatives such as benzodiazepines into street acquired opioids. Between April 11–24th, 2020 Toronto's Drug Checking Services (April 25 – May 8, 2020, Centre on Drug Policy Evaluation, 2020) reported that 38% of tested fentanyl samples contained benzodiazepine-related drugs. Heavy sedation and unresponsiveness caused by benzodiazepines are presenting more challenges in identifying and responding to overdoses.

When preventing overdose and disease transmission for people who use drugs, harm reduction strategies can be a literal lifesaver. Harm reduction practices decrease the negative impacts of drug use by providing clean supplies to prevent disease transmission, teaching practical overdose prevention strategies and by providing safe injection and overdose prevention sites. As COVID-19 precautions have closed many harm reduction services and drug checking sites decrease hours of service, users are given fewer options to access clean drug works and overdose prevention supports. Due to the decrease in accessible harm reduction services, we could possibly see an increase of communicable disease transmission and overdose during the COIVD-19 pandemic.

While working with agencies that primarily support people experiencing homelessness, it is apparent that the intersecting circumstances of homelessness and substance use generate a range of factors that influence health and safety. People who use drugs and experience homelessness have a particularly difficult time physically distancing themselves from others as the need to acquire food, shelter and substances can be dependent on daily physical interactions with community agencies and community members. This may pose a higher risk of contracting or transmitting COIVD-19 for this population.

According to The City of Toronto's *COVID-19 Response for People Experiencing Homelessness*, 1,850 respites, hotels and temporary housing units are to be available by April 30.2020 (CITY of Toronto COVID response, pp 1, 2020). However, only people who access the shelter system are eligible for these units. Many people experiencing homelessness do not access the shelter system for a number of reasons, such as transportation, shelter restrictions prohibiting intoxication, mental illness, or congested shelter spaces. During COVID 19, overcrowding and the fear of contracting the virus within these densely populated facilities have many feeling safer sleeping on the streets. For these individuals, the closing of local businesses, libraries and community centers has made it increasingly difficult to use a washroom, wash their hands or just get a glass of water.

Understanding the various health implications and safety concerns for people who use drugs unveils some of the challenges this population may face during COIVD-19. While safe drug supplies are becoming harder to find and drug checking sites become harder to access, the rates of drug mixing and overdose are set to rise. For IV drug users, lack of access to harm reduction supplies such as needles may lead to higher rates of HIV and Hepatitis C through sharing drug works. The overcrowding or shelters and lack of access to sanitizing stations for people experiencing homelessness leave many without armor to fight the virus in their communities.

During social crises, public health emergencies and economic downturns, people who are chronically facing marginalization are disproportionately impacted. Societal and government response to such crises are not typically focused on the needs and specific circumstances of those living on the margins of society. The long-term consequences of this pandemic will undoubtedly include a further marginalization of drug users. The public image of drug users is very unfavorable, with stereotypes and stigmatization that will be hard to shift. In reality, long before there was COVID-19, Canada was in the midst of an opiate crisis, another type of public health emergency that did not garner the kind of political mobilization we now see with this middle class crisis and associated economic doom and gloom. Drug users include people from all walks of life and all ages; youth, their families and their communities are impacted significantly. We must ensure that our response to the current pandemic does not unfold by simply sidelining and forgetting about a preexisting public health crisis. Instead, our pandemic response should include programs that deliver a safe supply of prescribed opioids directly to people experiencing dependency. Partnering with local harm reduction services, more drop-ins and addiction based programing, and of course advocacy for shelter and housing supports while supporting accessibility to general health care should be priorities. With the overlapping issues of COVID-19, the opioid epidemic and the housing crisis, it is evident that we have a lot of work to do to support people living with multiple barriers in Toronto and in other major urban centers across North America.

References

Centre on Drug Policy Evaluation. (2020). *Results from samples checked by Toronto's drug checking service: April 25–May 8, 2020.* https://cdpe.org/news/#

City of Toronto. (2020). *City of Toronto COVID-19 response for people experiencing homelessness.* PowerPoint. https://www.toronto.ca/home/media-room/backgrounders-other-resources/backgrounder-city-of-toronto-covid-19-response-for-people-experiencing-homelessness/

A Unique Experience

Jordan Risidore

Covid-19 has been a truly unique experience. It feels quite surreal, to have to watch the world pass by through my window. Connecting with friends and loved ones is now done virtually as there is the ever-present fear that I will become one of the many infected or or even worse transmit this invisible assassin to another, a thought I could not bear. Never have I thought so intently on the fate of humanity and the long and short-term ramifications for us all. When will this all be over? How will we transition back to normalcy? These questions add to my list of worries about what is already going on globally, in our communities, and how this will impact my already unclear future. These are but a few of my many thoughts that, as of late, never cease.

When I was young, my mother always used to tell me to be thankful for what I have. This was a tall ask as I grew up economically disadvantaged and did not see myself as being fortunate. On what seemed like a daily basis, she would have to remind me that I had clothes on my back, food on my plate, and a roof over my head. This type of thinking eventually became ingrained in my head and has lingered ever since. As a young Black male, I have never found myself identifying with privilege, but the pandemic has been somewhat of a humbling experience. For the first time in my life I see myself as possessing privilege. My income has not been disrupted, as I have a good job that I can do from the comfort of my living room, my fridge is always stocked, I have an amazing partner whom I share an apartment with, and my support system is being amplified. I feel thankful for every breath I take. However, I acknowledge that many people's lives are in shambles. For that reason, I am truly worried about how others are faring considering people are forced to go to work and put themselves at risk to survive. Also, we have been ordered to remain indoors and only leave our homes when it is necessary to utilize essential services such as grocery stores and health-care related services. The world is temporarily on halt, and despite these necessary restrictions, some people are worried more about the economy than human life. These folks refuse to comply with the new rules being implemented to deter risk and spread of infection. This is concerning.

Family life, for many, has been drastically altered. With schools closed, parents have become teachers, chefs, coaches, and counselors. Some parents have lost their job. Larger families are cooped up and have less time for personal space. For many youths, school is a place of safety, and then suddenly, this haven has been removed. I cannot fathom how the children, who may be at greater risk of abuse, are coping while stuck at home. They cannot leave, hangout with friends, or seek support like they could before. Will this lead to further trauma? I imagine families struggling to get along, becoming irritable, or struggling to cope with mental health related issues. I also think about individuals who are in an abusive relationship and are increasingly at risk of being in danger. I commend the creative things that are being done to help victims of domestic abuse. For instance, I have seen people on Facebook cleverly posting statuses that say "text me these ingredients…. And I will know you are in trouble and will call the authorities". Even at the worst of times, there are good people willing to help. Similarly, there are several students and health care professionals stepping up to the front line and volunteering with the influx of need from 'kids help phone'. I hope that people continue to step up and attempt to take this time to create solidarity and uplift each other as opposed to the toxicity emanating from selfishness. We are all in the same boat.

Unfortunately, being a young Black male who has been conditioned to be hyperaware of social injustices normally, I have noticed an increase in discrimination that provokes a concerning trail of thought. For instance, how might Black communities be impacted? Well, for one, many Black folks are less likely to have a job that allows them to work from home, increasing their vulnerability due to the virus and lack of access to healthcare resources. This has created a crisis within a crisis for many marginalized communities.

Xenophobia has become more prevalent as people are blaming the Asian community for the outburst of this pandemic. Also disheartening as a member of a marginalized community is seeing the needs of the homeless being swept under the rug. Just as concerning are the people who complain about how the liquor stores are unnecessarily staying open. If places such as these were closed, addicts who suffer life-threatening withdrawal would possibly suffer dire consequences - many fail to understand the complexities and needs that come with alcoholism.

It would be my hope that the severity of the pandemic would bring people together, but I do not see this occurring. Rather, I see bureaucracy reinforcing who deserves support and who is left to fend for themselves. I have been trying to reframe the way I perceive the pandemic. One of the main rules throughout the pandemic has been to commit to social distancing. Although, I think this is problematic, and reinforces the importance of language and how we should model language appropriately. The term social distancing should be renamed as physical distancing. During this pandemic we should refrain from sacrificing our social connections and abide by the essential 'physical' restrictions currently implemented. We should be uniting and working together to get through this, as we are all connected. I am hoping that the new normal will encompass systemic changes, an increased empathy within societies and culturally responsive policies in place moving forward. Ultimately, I hope we can maximize our greatest potential – solidarity.

COVID-19 and Youth in Detention

William Rowe

The COVID-19 pandemic has fueled behavior changes in numerous areas at a breathtaking pace, and in ways that are having immediate and perhaps more long-term consequences. Two public health messages: Stay at home when possible and social distance when staying home is not possible are especially challenging to confined populations such as youth in detention or corrections facilities. On any given day there are more than 48,000 youth confined in facilities away from home in the United States. While these numbers have declined significantly in the past 20 years, they still represent a large number of youth at high risk of coronavirus infection. Many jurisdictions spurred on by the health crisis are rushing to see which youth in their care can safely be supervised at home or in a homelike setting in the community. This is especially true for youth who have committed status offenses or revocations. The move toward greater use of diversion programs and least restrictive environments has been a trend in youth justice for some time. Some well-designed and evidence-based diversion programs have shown less than 10% reoffense rates following the successful completion of these programs. The research on juvenile incarceration indicates that it fails to reduce recidivism and in many cases is counterproductive, with more youth likely to reoffend after an institutional stay.

Is it possible that this short-term emergency response to COVID-19 could point the way to long-term benefits? The vast majority of youth who enter the school to prison pipeline come from distressed and underresourced home settings, be they urban or rural. In addition, they are overrepresented by black and brown populations, who have been shown to suffer higher infection and death rates from COVID-19. A positive outcome from the pandemic could be the development of more creative ways to maintain these youths in their homes and neighborhoods by identifying and building on the inherent strengths in those neighborhoods, including people, programs, and facilities. For a number of years, I worked with a community development corporation in a neighborhood historically referred to as Suitcase City. The name originated because poor residents moved there for the low rent but did not unpack their suitcases. They knew they would be evicted eventually, leading to a continuously unstable neighborhood. Over a 20-year period, the community development corporation managed to build a large multipurpose community center, a general education diploma (GED) high school, A Junior Achievement Center, a county-sponsored community health center, a social service center, and an employment center, to name a few. In essence, this transformed a blighted neighborhood into a main street community. Numerous health, social, and educational programs were established and staffed primarily by people from the neighborhood. By centering programs and services in the neighborhood with people from the neighborhood, trust capital was built to a level where even local gangs declared the community center and the other service centers neutral territory.

The longer-term economic effects of the pandemic will mean diminished funding for all services, including youth corrections. The cost of policing, the courts, and especially residential care are reason enough to continue the reforms that have been underway and to concentrate efforts in developing and supporting resources at the most local levels at churches, community centers, and neighborhood associations. The worldwide protests that have been sparked by George Floyd's death in police custody and the misuse of nonlocal police forces employing military tactics to deal with the protesters greatly expand the distrust of institutional authority that already exists in these distressed neighborhoods. The distrust is exacerbated as we see powerful and connected white men being released to their homes to serve their sentences to protect them from coronavirus infection while poor black and brown inmates remain incarcerated in facilities with some of the highest infection rates. The Marshall Project reported on the plight of juvenile lifers, who now have the possibility of a sentence review (which in most cases will take years), but are currently living in prison facilities, some of which have more than 80% infection rates.

The mass removal and incarceration of black and brown men and with the privatization of prisons have left many of those neighborhoods without the human and social capital needed to build and maintain nurturing social structures. Funds spent in locations, often far from the neighborhoods where the residents come from and will be returning to, would be better directed toward prevention, diversion, and mental health programs located in those very neighborhoods. Some law enforcement agencies claim they have had to expand their budgets to deal with social problems like child abuse, school, and family violence. Most working in human services welcomed cooperating and coordinating with law enforcement to deal with these situations; however, the unintended consequence has been that children and youth more often have their first out-of-home authority experience with a uniformed officer, who may or may not embrace the values of dignity, respect, support, and self-determination. Many of those law enforcement agencies aggressively competed for the contracts and budgets that accompany the administration and delivery of those services. They were often successful partly because they prioritized safe communities over healthy communities. Safe communities was a more supportable concept especially by taxpayers who did not live in those neighborhoods.

The long-term management of COVID-19 is likely to include practices such as staying home and social distancing with a smaller circle of trusted people so that children and youth can receive services from home, as is the current practice. Then perhaps we can continue those community based services long term if we rightly focus on promoting healthy communities, those with strengths-based neighborhood associations, strong schools, high quality health care, and mental health services—the long list of what makes a good neighborhood "good."

Renewed Grammars of Care: A(n Abbreviated) Case for the End of "the Service Provider"

Juanita Stephen and Nataleah Hunter-Young

> Such far-reaching notions of what could be were the fruit of centuries of mutual aid, which was organized in stealth and paraded in public view.
>
> Saidiya Hartman, *The Anarchy of Colored Girls Assembled in a Riotous Manner*

> ... some ancient ritual we remembered from nowhere and no one.
>
> Dionne Brand, The Blue Clerk, *Verso 55*

We write this as both them and us; the carers and the cared for; positioned as, at, and beyond the limits of social compassion and state care. We offer this reflection to the collective as a provocation and invite you to read it as such.

Neighbours are readying their pots, pans, and other noisemakers for the daily celebration of health care workers *on the front lines* of the COVID-19 pandemic. Social media reminds us to thank grocery store staff, truck drivers, and other laborers newly named *essential.* As they did in wartime, ribbons wrap trees across North America offering silent gratitude to these workers for their service and their sacrifice. The comparisons to military personnel are both convenient and familiar; it is how we have been taught great threats are eliminated. They fight for our wellbeing, our safety. Some sacrifice and some are sacrificed for the benefit of all. It is their now *essential* job. We are to do our part by staying inside, distancing ourselves from the virus and the vulnerable. The ribbons and noisy applause welcome silent sacrifice and drown out sounds of protest. When we listen, what other sounds does sacrifice make?

We have heard governments across Canada mobilize the language of *essential* worker in lieu of the more accurate *sacrificial* worker. To use the latter would demand an acknowledgement that a segment of the population has been designated to take on disproportionate risk[1] to maintain an uneven and racist economy for the preservation of mostly white, middle

[1]Our frame is indebted to Christina Sharpe whose "thinking aloud" on social media about the (re)distribution of risk has helped us greatly in finding language for this "moment".

class lives. Likewise, our governments have commodified care so as to position service providers as "professionalized caregivers." In this framework, our governments situate service providers as the gatekeepers representing the boundary and limit of care. Our social order places the responsibility of providing care (noun) on the helping industry. Surely any practice can be done carefully (adverb) but to care (verb) as a public service and care (noun) as a commodity are consigned to the domain of nurses, doctors, personal support workers, paramedics, social workers, child and youth care practitioners and others. Each level of government transfers payment to agencies (for profit and otherwise) to administer care. And when endowed with this responsibility, agency staff become *the service provider* upon whom the provision of care rests. Saidiya Hartman warns of the state's illusions of care in Wayward Lives, Beautiful Experiments. Hartman (2019) writes, "the reformers used words like 'improvement' and 'social betterment' and 'protection,' but no one was fooled". In school the reformers, otherwise known as the service providers, learn to understand themselves as separate from the cared for and that only by this separation should they provide care to another. Only through this distancing, this ordering, are they *able* to care for another. In fact, it is this prescribed separation that defines the social conditions for service providers to perform care. For Black and Indigenous peoples, this pandemic has reinforced a constructed binary between service provider and service user. We wonder what it might look like to resist this separation; to refuse the division that has always been complicated by those of us who traverse the imagined chasm between service provision and service use.

Though the language of *care* is often used, service provision frequently fails to meet "what is necessary for the health, welfare, maintenance, and protection of someone or something."[2] The service provider of state-administered financial aid, for example, becomes instead an interface between the state and the service user, embodying and enacting the will of the state with little discretion for the person and their needs. The violence of prisons and policing, replete with service provision, forestalls the presence of care, though it may persist laterally. The service provider – the reformer – cannot make a death space a life space. To make life, instead, we must "inhabit a deviant set of relations not only to the state but also to one another" (Hwang, 2019, p. 561). To preserve life we must co-construct care. Calling for the end of *the service provider* is a move away from a system that identifies the carers as only a segment of our population and toward a framework that insists on caring as a way of being for us all. It

[2]Oxford dictionary's definition of "care."

imagines the possibility of mutual aid; care outside of professionalized (and credentialized) industry.

Despite widespread closures amid physical distancing, we witness individuals mobilizing whatever they have to demonstrate care – sewing masks, donating and delivering groceries, cooking and sharing food for sustenance and love. Our collective need to be cared for – and to offer care – has led many to stream dance classes, concerts, lectures, workshops, guided meditations, weddings, birthdays and funerals for groups seeking new ways to celebrate, commune, protest, and grieve. To think strategies anew is familiar to Black and Indigenous peoples, for whom the state regularly does not (provide) care. In that sense, reimagining social relationships to care only requires each other. For many of us, an ethic of care is already foundational to our ways of being. Traditions of reciprocity and collectivity have sustained us in the face of genocide and exile; as we were forced onto ships and fruitless lands; as our homes were demolished and we were relegated to reserves, townships, and tenements. Mutual aid and lateral care have spelled survival for those of us who think in terms of "we" rather than "I" because *we* have always been sacrificed by white supremacy in the name of capital. As Lee Maracle (2015) teaches, "the fastest road to healing is to metaphorically express the memory in poetic form and draw lessons from it" (p. 36). We recognize that our best chance for wellness is in *re-membering* to take and give care to each other.

We call for *the service provider* to no longer be considered, or to consider themselves, the keepers of care. We call for the dissolution of the service provider-service user binary in favor of a renewed grammar of care that insists on the emotional, material and risk investment from all members of society into one another and ourselves.

References

Hartman, S. (2019). *Wayward lives, beautiful experiments: Intimate histories of social upheaval.* Norton & Company, Inc.

Hwang, R. (2019). Deviant care for deviant futures: QTBIPoC radical relationalism as mutual aid against carceral care. *Transgender Studies Quarterly*, *6*(4), 559–578. https://doi.org/10.1215/23289252-7771723

Maracle, L. (2015). *Memory serves: Oratories.* (S. Kamboureli, Ed.). NeWest Press.

Coronavirus and Youth

Curren Warf

Pandemics at first glance can seem like the great equalizer, affecting young and old, affluent and poor, locally born and migrants. The impacts of the coronavirus pandemic belie this impression and the tragic consequences of intergenerational inequities are plain to see. The historic legacy of poverty and marginalization leaves large populations of youth with very high levels of vulnerability and grossly disproportionate risks of infection and death, in particular those with unstable and crowded housing, in residential care or group homes, youth detention or shelters.

The short-term consequences for children and youth will be, and already have been, grave.

In the United States, schools have been closed and it remains uncertain if students will return to school in the near future. For children and youth, school provides a key social environment, and the relationships with teachers and other school staff, as well as their peers, are formative in their development, especially for young people from stressed family environments. The cancelation of school removes children and youth from their natural social community. Youth and children who are out of school for prolonged periods, in addition to reduced socialization opportunities, may experience lasting impact on education and preparation for employment preparation.

The practice of 'shelter in place', though necessary to meet public health objectives of reducing the prevalence of coronavirus infections, has a potentially negative effect on the social and family relationships necessary for healthy development. Creative attempts at continuing education in the midst of the pandemic that rely heavily on online courses may exclude those youth without computers or online access.

The economic impact on families through parental loss of employment and income is profound and will further threaten the resources available to support many children and youth. The unprecedented growth in unemployment and economic insecurity with consequent food and housing insecurity creates a compelling need to find work locally or in more distant urban centers. 'Shelter in place', a reasonable if difficult approach for people with homes, can for those without stable homes increase the need to move and risk disseminating the infection. Already stressed parents may have no resources to enable them to care for children at home when they face the compelling need of continuing to go to work.

The disproportionate impact of the pandemic on low-income communities, in particular African American and Indigenous communities in the US, further challenges many parents' ability to provide safe, stable and loving environments for their children. Mortality and prevalence rates of coronavirus are grossly disproportionate for African Americans and Indigenous people, related to the prevalence of preexisting health conditions and other factors.

Without large-scale government support for housing and food, the pandemic is destined to create further desperation. The economic pressures of sustaining shelter-in-place will challenge the capacity to sustain public health interventions and lead desperate youth and parents to seek out employment, food and shelter, probably followed by second and third waves of the pandemic. Youth entering the economy with gig jobs, part-time service jobs, in coffee shops and restaurants generally have low wages, long hours and no benefits, including no health insurance.

Online communication and employment may set the stage for great changes in the economy at least for some of the more educated youth, so that their work and career expectations may be very different than prior generations. These may be changes that the younger generation may be better equipped to adjust to although this remains to be seen.

The disproportionate vulnerability of the elderly to lethal consequences of the infection removes key figures from the lives of children and youth, and their parents. This loss of key family members will be the first major loss in the lives of many young people. There may be ripple effects on the emotional health of their parents as well who suffer the loss of their parents, siblings and others as well as a disconnection from their family and cultural histories. High vulnerability based on age and existing medical conditions, further erodes natural social support from extended families for youth including parents, grandparents, community seniors and leaders and threatens continuity of culture.

The discontinuation of public gatherings that support the continuation of cultures including religious and spiritual ceremonies, youth sports, wakes and funerals, group holiday events, public athletic events and musical concerts threaten to leave a lasting disconnection of youth from their cultures. Longer term consequences for children, families and youth may include new challenges to sustaining intergenerational cultural practices and traditions potentially changing the sense of identity for the upcoming generations.

Societies without universal health care put youth and their parents at an extraordinarily high level of threat, in particular the United States. Those adults and their children who work and reside in the US, particularly low-income agricultural workers providing essential services of food production, garment workers and many service workers, receive no employment-related health insurance or other benefits, and exist under threat of deportation if they complain. It is a deep irony that migrant workers and their children who are at once undocumented (or 'illegal') are simultaneously designated as 'essential workers' for food production.

The medical complications of the coronavirus infection include the presentation in children and youth of the previously rare but serious Kawasaki syndrome and toxic shock syndrome, blood coagulation risks with central nervous system strokes, and chronic pulmonary symptoms in survivors. Focus of the medical system on addressing the sickest and most high-risk patients in tertiary care facilities, may deter emphasis and funding from effective public health approaches to prevention and early intervention.

Lack of planning and preparation, especially in the US, with the rejection of scientific public health and medical advice and failed leadership at a national level, creates confusion and puts large numbers of families and youth at risk for serious illness or death. The lack of planning, politicization and rejection of international collaboration has placed gratuitous obstacles in the path of developing an urgently needed effective vaccine.

It is difficult to see much in the way of advantages, except to note that many children and youth can be surprisingly resilient even under the most difficult circumstances. Loss of loved ones is a part of life, and young people can survive, learn and grow in the context of adverse experiences particularly if there is a broader family and social network involved. If the shared loss can bring communities and extended family members together for renewed focus on the well-being of their children, the groundwork for the emergence of a stronger support and broader social and family support system may be laid.

There is no assurance that even with control of the pandemic, still a year or several years away under the best of circumstances, that there will be a return to the past social practices regarding work and employment. What will the 'New Normal' be? This is a compelling question that remains unanswered.

The threats are very real. The current pandemic with coronavirus may well destabilize core elements of the established order and leave in its wake challenges to every modern economy. The willingness of the political leadership to embrace difficult but effective public health interventions, the provision of medical care to all residents and migrants without the threat of deportation or detention, the rapid reduction and release of incarcerated people who do not represent a significant threat of violence, especially youth in detention, attention to housing stabilization, food stability, education, employment and/or job preparation can provide compassionate and healing opportunities. Young people will inevitably face their own new challenges.

Navigating the COVID-19 Pandemic: The Future of Children and Young People

Khadijah Williams

Many of the young people I work with have experienced trauma, neglect and abandonment and they may have a more difficult time dealing with the uncertainty, threats to life, detachment and isolation associated with the pandemic. Messages of hope can appear to be useless with all the negativity surrounding us, which only adds to their existing narratives of loss and despair, abuse and neglect. This makes the work of caregivers, youth workers and social care providers more challenging.

As a result, I would think that the adults around them need to be positive, demonstrate faith, be honest about their concerns and challenges, be patient and willing to engage the young people so that their interpretation of reality is understood and contextualized. The spaces in which we come into contact with children and young people must be supportive of their development and more inclusive of adults who are willing to share their power with them. That is, recognize their contributions, their resilience, their concerns and their realities. Furthermore, schools, churches, business places, and communities, should have the infrastructure to support the staff, including the materials, resources and technologies that are required for mutually beneficial exchanges with children and young people. Therefore, when communicating with children and young people our language should include messages of:

Faith and being fearless: Many biblical stories exist where Jesus taught us about the importance of having faith. For the less religiously inclined, there are personal testimonies that can be shared about having faith and the outcomes of such faith. It is a critical time to tell stories of faith – to help young people understand beyond their virtual worlds and movies as well as their own tragic episodes that stories with bad beginnings can have happy endings and result in more progressive and empowered persons.

Resilience and agency: Messages about overcoming struggles and being resilient are even more relevant for young people throughout these times. There are many stories of civilizations that have survived massacres, slavery, world wars, famines, and other natural and man-made disasters. I have no doubt that the young people who will survive this tragedy will be stronger and more spiritually enlightened, having lived through this period that will certainly alter how we live. Helping young people to see that they have the capacity to influence positive changes in small things is necessary so it becomes second nature for them to contribute positively in the bigger things, such as when there is a crisis.

Creativity and Innovation: The future will require more thought about how to survive with limited resources and greater demands from people. Young people will be required to think more critically and to be practical with a high degree of technical competence. This crisis has tested our ability to be self-sufficient, creative and resourceful. Having technical competence in various skill areas will surely be important. Important is also the ability to empathize and be emotionally intelligent so that they can think ahead about other people's needs, thereby being insightful, proactive and productive.

Being selfless: Developing a deep sense of community spirit, volunteerism and social skills cannot be emphasized enough. Despite technological advancements that facilitate physical distancing of people, the skills that bring people together (virtually or otherwise) will continue to be fundamental skills for survival. Redefining what it means to be sociable and how to act collectively and understanding how to provide emotional, psychological or physical assistance to others, will certainly be an outcome of this new pandemic experience. Now more than ever we are learning that 'no man is an island' – that we are interdependent beings, eager to make connections and desirous of fulfilling our purpose. Young people will thrive with more collectivism, less individualism.

The land and its people: Agriculture an important venture

Given my current position, located in rural Jamaica in the midst of the beautiful rain forest, managing an agriculture school with young people, I am inspired to think about the important role of agriculture in safeguarding humanity and preserving health and well-being. Its role in the lives of young people is still to be explored fully. Social-agriculture as we call it, acknowledges the important relationship between the land and the psychosocial and socio-emotional aspects of people. It provides a space for self-reflection, self-discovery, building confidence and instilling hope. Land exposes us to the elements of wind, earth, sun, water, animals, vegetation and even fire. The connection with the land has been therapeutic in itself for many young people, and also staff, at my school. Agronomy has taught us the importance of nurturing roots in order to thrive, the importance of removing parasites which stagnate growth. The bees at our school's apiary unit have taught us the importance of interdependence, working together as a team to get more accomplished and that there is more strength in numbers.

Nurturing the earth demands silence, meditation and undivided attention, which is also good for the soul. Through this practice, we learn to quiet our minds, focus and discover self. We learn to plant a seed, till the soil, feed and care for animals. The results speak a language of hope – that there is life – that there is truth – that with actions of faith, we can reap and survive.

For those who follow the argument that animals are a key source of many bacteria and viruses that transmit to humans and what this can mean for the future of agriculture, I must admit that although this may be true, learning the biosecurity measures that should be adhered to in this business should be taken more seriously. In fact, based on my prior knowledge, having participated in several training sessions conducted by experts in this area, my preparation for the current pandemic was facilitated. Sanitization, personal hygiene, boosting the immune system and using personal protective equipment (PPE) as the everyday common language at my school has indeed been useful. Additionally, we need to apply best practices when it comes to agriculture in order that we can eat healthy food. So, encouraging young people to apply the various technologies that support food production and preserving the land is another very positive step.

We should continue to seek answers that will advance our thinking about the meaning of the present crisis as it relates to our children and young people and their future. The future as we see it today demands a new way of thinking about many things. Although the answers may be unclear at the moment, the need to inspire hope for young minds to be nurtured and our future to be secure is very clear.

Galvanizing Solidarity Through Chaos: Policing, Surveillance and the Impact of COVID-19 on Black Canadian Youth

Keisha Evans and Lesa Francis

In *Dark Matters: On the Surveillance of Blackness*, Simone Browne writes, "Racializing surveillance is a technology of social control where surveillance practices, policies, and performances concern the production of norms pertaining to race and exercise a power to define what is in or out of place." Browne powerfully articulates how Black people have always been burdened by the white gaze. Since the era of slavery, Black people have been under constant observation, monitoring, and scrutiny by those who are in positions of power and privilege. The present novel coronavirus (COVID-19) pandemic provides for a convenient cover for evermore intensive and overt surveillance practices impacting Black people disproportionately and further accelerating inequities and injustices in the relationships between Black people and policymakers and the criminal justice system. This surveillance draws its roots from racist practices entrenched within laws that allow the police and the criminal justice system to abuse their power and exert control. The same dynamics that shape the systemically racist application of laws also mold the policing practices and policies designed to contain the current pandemic. COVID-19 will exacerbate an already racist law enforcement system and further complicate the dynamic between police and Black Canadian youth. These troubling issues will create an urgent need for Black Canadians to work even closer together to galvanize through the ensuing chaos.

We are experiencing a societal transformation, a time of uncertainty, facing something most of us have never encountered before—a global health pandemic. The government has mandated that everyone "stay at home" and practice social distancing to minimize the spread of the potentially deadly coronavirus. Those caught disregarding these orders are subjected to fines or charges. Maintaining these newly implemented rules on movement and social distancing has created an increase in police presence, especially in marginalized communities where covert surveillance measures have been in place for some time. This increased surveillance puts Black youth at greater risk of imposed and coercive interventions, this time under the seemingly legitimate guise of public safety. Across Canada, in comparison to their white counterparts, Black youth are disproportionately being targeted, getting fines, and arrested under claims that they are not following the social distancing orders (Bain et al., 2020). For example, the police were called on four Black youth sitting on a bench outside of a Scarborough shelter where they reside. The police indicated that they received reports that the youth were not socially distancing. It was necessary for staff to intervene on behalf of the youth to prevent an escalation and an issuance of fines. The youth felt that they were racially profiled and found the encounter traumatizing and were convinced had they been white the police would not have been called.

In addition to the implications of social distancing and stay-at-home directives, Black Canadian youth are also impacted by health officials' suggestion that we wear facial masks as a means of protection. Due to systemic anti-Black racism and the ongoing criminalization of Black skin, wearing facial masks in public while gathered in groups of more than five could potentially be seen as menacing, threatening, and criminal under the white gaze through which Black people are viewed as dangerous and fearsome. This is not far-fetched - the Ontario Human Rights Commission reports that "between 2013 and 2017, a Black person in Toronto was nearly 20 times more likely than a White person to be involved in a fatal shooting by the Toronto Police Service" (OHRC, 2018). Black youth have been criminalized and profiled by police officers and even private citizens simply for wearing hoodies, both in Canada and in the United States. This fear and criminalization of Black people make it more likely that police will be called on Black youth who cover their faces in accordance with the public health recommendations, leading to increased interactions between police and Black youth and potential involvement in the justice system. While the new Emergency Order in Council allows police officers to demand identifying information if they have reasonable grounds to believe that any order has been violated, the directive around face masks also demonstrates how obeying these orders can be equally troublesome for Black youth. They have to choose between protecting their health or risk being racially profiled.

The physical and mental health risks that Black Canadian youth will endure when interacting with police during COVID-19 cannot be overstated. Working with youth who are homeless, live with mental health concerns, reside in shelters, or live in priority neighborhoods where police presence has increased, we have seen the effects that these orders have, especially on young Black males. It is necessary to advocate in these instances to reduce the possibility of criminalizing these youth.

However, when concerned parents and youth advocates question these inequitable policies and policing tactics, the response is that they are necessary to protect the general public from contracting the virus. The new orders and the enforcement that supports them has left us paralyzed with fear, not only for the youth that we work with, but also for our own Black sons. Black lives have been imperiled by this pandemic, not only by the virus but the policies put in place to eradicate it. The criminal justice system has found an additional way to over-police us, and we expect to see a surge in the race-based data on the over-surveillance and over-policing in Black communities. The implications are increased racial profiling and harassment toward Black youth, who will lose their ability to move around society without confidence that the police will serve and protect them equally.

Acknowledging that the pandemic has adverse effects on the protection of Black youth in no way detracts from the experience of other racialized communities that have distinctive issues with profiling and other human rights violations. However, the negative effects of the COVID-19 pandemic on Black people seems to be, in part, an extension of poor policing policies and structural and institutional anti-Black racism that made it a political and social norm to position Black youth as dubious and nefarious in their movements long before this pandemic began. As members of this community, we know first-hand that we are surveilled at disproportionate rates. This is the reason why organizations such as Color of Poverty-Color of Change have sent out a call for human rights oversight of government responses to the COVID-19 pandemic. However, due to the lack of trust we already have when it comes to policing Black bodies, we are certain that in the aftermath of COVID-19, the long term effect is that fear and racism will heighten instances of human rights violations toward Black people, particularly our youth.

But we are not powerless. In the past, despite the over-policing and the criminalization of our basic movements (e.g. driving while Black), we have managed to individually and collectively overcome injustices, empower each other, and unite as a community. We have held hands through freedom marches, prayed together in silent protest of unfair and inequitable policy making, and rallied together through the tragedies of police brutality on Black lives. In spite of the iniquitous targeting of Black communities in Canada (and elsewhere), we still find ways to overcome this adversity. In the long term, it will be vital for us to continue to stand together in solidarity, building stronger community connections, empowering and advocating for our youth, and supporting their mental health and emotional stability, notwithstanding unprecedented pandemics and policing tactics.

References

Bain, B., Dryden, O., & Walcott, R., (2020, April 20). Coronavirus discriminates against Black lives through surveillance, policing and the absence of health data. *The Conversation.* https://theconversation.com/coronavirus-discriminates-against-black-lives-through-surveillance-policing-and-the-absence-of-health-data-135906

Browne, S., (2015). *Dark matters: On the surveillance of blackness.* Duke University Press.

Ontario Human Rights Commission. (2018, November). *A Collective Impact: Interim report on the inquiry into racial profiling and racial discrimination of Black persons by the Toronto Police Service.* http://www.ohrc.on.ca/en/public-interest-inquiry-racial-profiling-and-discrimination-toronto-police-service/collective-impact-interim-report-inquiry-racial-profiling-and-racial-discrimination-black.

Index

For Product Safety Concerns and Information please contact our EU
representative GPSR@taylorandfrancis.com
Taylor & Francis Verlag GmbH, Kaufingerstraße 24, 80331 München, Germany

www.ingramcontent.com/pod-product-compliance
Ingram Content Group UK Ltd.
Pitfield, Milton Keynes, MK11 3LW, UK
UKHW052053230926
475702UK00025B/1151
* 9 7 8 1 0 3 2 2 2 7 4 9 8 *